Baby Ever After

Expanding Your Family After Postpartum Depression

Rebecca Fox Starr

ROWMAN & LITTLEFIELD
Lanham • Boulder • New York • London

Published by Rowman & Littlefield
A wholly owned subsidary of The Rowman & Littlefield Publishing Group, Inc.
4501 Forbes Boulevard, Suite 200, Lanham, Maryland 20706
www.rowman.com

6 Tinworth Street, London SE11 5AL, United Kingdom

British Library Cataloguing in Publication Information Available

Library of Congress Cataloging-in-Publication Data
Names: Fox Starr, Rebecca, 1985– author.
Title: Baby ever after : expanding your family after postpartum depression /
    Rebecca Fox Starr.
Description: Lanham : Rowman & Littlefield, [2020] | Includes bibliographical
    references and index. | Summary: "Choosing to have another baby after suffering
    from prenatal or postpartum depression can feel overwhelming and hopeless.
    It doesn't have to. Exploring existing options, complex emotions, and personal
    accounts, Rebecca Fox Starr takes readers on a thoughtful exploration of what
    choosing to have, or not have, another baby means to women and families"
    — Provided by publisher.
Identifiers: LCCN 2019038524 (print) | LCCN 2019038525 (ebook) |
    ISBN 9781538127377 (cloth) | ISBN 9781538127384 (epub)
Subjects: LCSH: Postpartum depression. | Pregnancy. | Families.
Classification: LCC RG852 .F68 2020 (print) | LCC RG852 (ebook) |
    DDC 618.7/6—dc23
LC record available at https://lccn.loc.gov/2019038524
LC ebook record available at https://lccn.loc.gov/2019038525

For Belle and Beau, the sweetest things I know

"It's not the weight you carry

but how you carry it—
books, bricks, grief—
it's all in the way
you embrace it, balance it, carry it

when you cannot, and would not,
put it down."

—Mary Oliver, from her poem "Heavy"

Contents

Acknowledgments

I know words, and I love words, but I simply do not have the words to express my gratitude for this book and for all of the people who have made it possible. While my journey with severe prenatal and postpartum anxiety and depression was devastating, I am also, in many ways, so grateful that it happened to me. It allowed me to find, and now use, my voice in an effort to help others.

Once again, I give my most sincere thanks to my amazing literary agent, Renée C. Fountain, president of Gandolfo Helin & Fountain Literary Management. I am blown away by what we have been able to accomplish since we started working together, more than half a decade ago, and that is thanks to you, R. Thank you for believing in me, for always going to bat for me, and for turning my passion into printed pages. Thank you to Italia Gandolfo and the rest of the Gandolfo Helin & Fountain community; your support has been astounding.

I am so grateful for my incredible editor at Rowman & Littlefield, Suzanne Staszak-Silva. Suzanne, you have turned my dreams into reality, and I am so inspired by your strength, determination, and generosity of spirit. You have given me more confidence than you'll ever know, and I can only hope that these two books are the first (and second!) of many together. I must also give a huge thanks to Patricia Stevenson, the editor who held my hand through my entire first publication process, as well as this one, and who brought me over the finish line. I am so grateful for Deborah Justice, the amazing copyeditor who so elegantly polished this book and caught me every time I repeated myself, which is a miraculous feat. Thank you to the entire Rowman & Littlefield team, as I believe we are changing lives for the better. I must also thank Ronnie Maier, indexer extraordinaire, who did for me what I could not and who allows my readers to find all of the "pineapple" passages with ease.

I do not know how to properly thank my treatment-team members, as they are gifted, magnificent doctors and my personal rock stars. Dr. S and Dr. B, you are my heroes. I can say, with conviction, that I literally would not be here today without you. Thank you for pushing me to grow, nurturing me through the subsequent growing pains, and sharing your brilliance with me each week. It took a long time to get this dream team together, but now that I have you, I will never let you go. Thank you to my OBGYN for helping me through my two healthy pregnancies and for the encouragement I needed for this exploration. Dr. G, you make babies each and every day, for women and for families, but I want to thank you for helping to make *me* into a version of Becca that I did not know I had in me. Speaking of world-class physicians, Dr. Schulman, you saved my life. You may be a neurologist, but by predicting my PPD and advocating for my care, you've become so much more to me. I will never stop giving you hugs when I visit your office.

On the topic of survival, this book has been made possible by the many courageous, strong, resilient, phenomenal women and men and sufferers who all identify as a part of this silent sodality. It is because of you that we are slowly stepping out of the dark shadow of the mental-health stigma, and you inspire me every single day. Thank you to the advocates, the activists, the doctors, the psychiatrists, the psychologists, the changemakers, the rabble-rousers, and those who have fought, tooth and nail, to survive. This is for those of you who have made it to the other side; this is for those who, tragically, have not. And to my tribe members in this crowd, you have changed me for good and *for good.*

This book would not exist without the exquisite courage and beautiful words shared by the women who have contributed to this text. Thank you to Brierley, Amanda, Nikki, Melissa, Becky, Hannah, and Samantha for so bravely unzipping yourselves and sharing your stories of postpartum depression, postpartum anxiety, postpartum psychosis, postpartum OCD, indecision, marriage, fear, survival, and a level of courage that I can only dream of being able to muster. Your vulnerability and honesty, in the face of great pain, is nothing short of miraculous. I will love and cherish each of you, always.

Once again, I thank you, my soul sisters. You each have a unique, unmatchable place in my heart. Thank you for loving me, even when I am not the easiest person to love. Thank you for tolerating me, even when I take up oh so much airspace. Thank you for never giving up on me and for modeling for me who I want to be. I love you, I appreciate you, and I am eternally and endlessly grateful to call you mine. You make me whole. You know who you are.

It is not often that you get to call a *New York Times*–bestselling author your book-writing mentor, but I am the luckiest because I also get to call her my sister. Emily, you are astounding. What you have accomplished in just three decades is mind blowing, but in many ways, with your preternatural diction and endless drive, I would expect nothing less. Em, I literally could not have done this without you. Thank you for being my guide and my sage, for the daily accountability check-ins, for sending me Levain cookies when I met my word count, and for forcing me to step back and take breaks. You made this daunting process doable (and even enjoyable!), and I love you more than you will ever, ever know. I am so glad that I wished for you, and I continue to wish for you every day so that you may get all that you deserve out of this life, which is so, so much.

Mom and Dad, when I say that I would not be here without you, I mean it in every single sense of the expression. You gave me life and then, in my darkest days, gave me the hope that I would find new life again. As with most things, you were right. I could not be more proud to be your daughter, as you are truly the two finest human beings I know. You are goodness personified, and you are the reason why I am a parent and also why I strive to be the best parent I can be. Your unwavering support, unconditional love, and consistent compassion allow me to be the person—and mother—I am today. I love you up to the moon and stars.

Kenny, Kenny, Kenny, where do I even begin? I am more in love with you today than I have ever been before or than I ever thought possible. You are my other (and better) half, my puzzle piece, and you continue to be my hero. Thank you for your exquisitely beautiful contribution to this book and for your exquisitely beautiful contributions to our life together. I am the luckiest girl alive to get to call you my "forever," and I am so blessed to have grown this family with you, in whatever form it ends up taking. I would be nothing without you. You are brilliant and brave and resilient and silly and steadfast and loyal and my home. That's how you look to me.

Belle and Beau, stars of *The Superkids Show* and my entire life: you two are the two most incredible humans I have ever known. You are so smart and kind and sensitive and caring and empathic and good, and I am so very proud to be your mommy. Thank you for helping me write this book and for making my heart grow bigger and bigger with love every single day. With each breath I take, I am filled with more and more adoration for you, and I will cherish you every single moment of my life. Thank you for loving each other so fiercely and for bringing Daddy and me along for your ride. Dancing through life with you two is the greatest joy one could ever know. You are precious love. You are inspiring. You are magic.

Prologue

As the ultrasound technician ran his wand across my pelvis, I stared at the grainy, black-and-white picture on the screen before me. This was not like any of my previous ultrasounds. I would not be holding my breath, waiting for a flickering heartbeat; I would not be asked whether I would like to know the sex; I would not see a tiny hand waving at me while tucked safely inside my womb. My womb was—and would forevermore be—empty. The tech was not looking for a yolk sac; he was examining my lymph nodes. He gently told me that he would be looking at my entire groin area, and when he reached my ovary and pressed down, I flinched, as it felt tender and swollen.

I made an offhand remark to him about how I must be ovulating.

"Wow, you know your body well! Look at this giant follicle you have here. Look at all of these eggs!"

I looked at the tiny grape-like structures swaying on the monitor, gazed at my husband, Kenny, who was sitting by my side, and tears formed in my eyes.

He held my hand. Kenny, more than anyone, knew why this was so hard for me—torturous.

I turned to him as the tech continued the examination.

"It's just so unfair," I cried. Sadness enveloped me, and tears dripped onto my hospital gown. "I just wish I had another chance. I wish we could try again."

I felt shattered. I still wanted another baby. I had never stopped wanting another baby.

Kenny looked at me, then back at the picture on the ultrasound machine's small, black screen, and then at me again, staring straight into my eyes.

"Maybe we can," he said, squeezing my hand a bit harder.

Maybe we can.

Part I

A HARD STORY

"Should I have another baby?"
"Should you have another baby?"
"How?"
"Why?"
"What makes me different from anyone else?"
"Why is my desire less valid?"

These are the questions that plague so many of us, no matter where we are from, what we have endured, or what stories are ours to tell. The question of family expansion is a universal one, with many people of childbearing age struggling to find "the right answer" to a question to which there is not just one.

Many of us have pictures in our minds, or dreams in our hearts, of what our families are supposed to look like, and when those expectations are violated, it can feel crushing. When things do not go as planned, whether physically or emotionally or situationally, where do we turn to find the answers? How do we move forward, and in what direction?

Women are expected to fit into certain archetypes, and, no matter what challenges we face, we are supposed to feel grateful—to count our blessings. While I am a champion of positive thinking, few things breed more guilt than when I am supposed to be enjoying something, or to be feeling content in a situation, yet cannot. In these situations, like in determining the size of my family, not only does society question me, but I also question myself. I had postpartum depression, but I am no different from a woman who had a postpartum hemorrhage or struggles with infertility or simply wants something out of life that is different from what she has. We all have beating hearts, though they don't beat to the exact same rhythm—the differences are simply in the details. In this book, I explore family

1

expansion after severe perinatal mood disorders, but, truly, this story could be about family expansion after *anything*. Prenatal and postpartum depression shape my personal story, but this topic, and these struggles, are collective. Here I am sharing as a way to help and encourage others and to provide individuals and families with a resource, filled with both emotions and options.

Postpartum depression and postpartum anxiety, two of the labels that I wear, are afflictions that have become increasingly visible in recent years. Celebrities and influencers are opening up about their battles with mental-health issues, clinicians are taking their patients more seriously when they express their postpartum woes, and, on a more intimate level, more and more women are opening up about their own struggles to their partners, to their families, to other women, and, most important, to themselves. When I first came out publicly with my (real-time) postpartum depression in February 2014, I was met with a lot of support and also many questions. I was a news story (literally) and, for many who followed my blog, the face of a sudden, debilitating mental-health disorder.

Now these stories are a dime a dozen, and my story is buried under weighty piles of narratives that are so much worse than my own. Of course, this situation is devastating for me, as I grieve the loss of so many members of my sisterhood; I survived and others did not. But the silver lining, though sometimes hard to see, is that my story is buried because people are now able to talk without shame about the subject that was once so scary—so stigmatized.

But despite all of the advancements in the treatment of perinatal mood disorders, and all of the increased exposure to mental-health issues, there is a wide chasm when it comes to our willingness to address the topic of family expansion after postpartum depression and our willingness to discuss other perinatal mood disorders. We have come so far, and yet there is hardly any data, online or in literature, about what a woman—or family—can do when they want to grow their family but are feeling (or met with) concern, doubt, and fear. In fact, when I try to search for answers on the Internet, the eighth hit that appears on Google.com is my own Instagram post on this topic.

This is why I write.

Expanding a family while recovering from, or coping with, mental illness is a topic that is extremely hard to research solely because of the lack of information. But as someone who has had some "on-the-job training" (so to speak) in the field of perinatal mood disorders, I have identified several ways in which I—or any mother—could consider family expansion after postpartum anxiety and depression.

Pregnancy after postpartum depression is a daunting idea, but it is one with which we wrestle (even going to extremes to achieve in some cases) nonetheless.

But what about the other options? In my exploration of how to expand my family after postpartum depression, whether the considerations were personal, professional, or found in the searching of my soul, I figured that, besides pregnancy, my options were adoption, surrogacy, and, importantly, not expanding my family at all. I also talk about the *middle place*, where many of us live—a place that is labeled "just not sure."

This book is an exploration. It is a tool to educate and to demystify the topic of family expansion after postpartum depression and to dive into each of the options I have laid out as deeply as I have been able to go. This book also touches on some of the hardest truths around perinatal mood disorders, including the effect that mental illness has on marriage and relationships, survivor's guilt, postpartum psychosis, and other things that typically fall under the "too taboo!" umbrella.

In some cases, I have rich insights from exquisite studies and clinical examples. In others, I am, in the words of Lady Gaga, "in the shallow."

In my own quest to explore family expansion after my own prenatal and postpartum anxiety and depression, I had nowhere to turn. There were no resources, and no one was talking about this sensitive issue. This book is, I hope, an antidote.

So whether you are struggling with the question of possibly expanding your family or wondering how to go about expanding your family, I have rolled up my sleeves and done a lot of the heavy lifting for you. I share the happy, the hard, and the hopeful so that you feel validated and seen and empowered. I unzip myself and make myself vulnerable so that you can stay whole. If I can help one of you in this process, then it is all worth it.

We are in this together. You are not alone. Let's do this.

1

My Shop Is Closed

Once upon a time, in the suburbs of Philadelphia, I met and married the boy who grew up around the corner, bought a couple of houses, had a couple of kids, and suffered from severe postpartum depression.

To be more accurate, I suffered from severe prenatal and postpartum anxiety and depression, and it almost took my life.

I am a survivor; I am one of the lucky ones. Through my experience I have learned that no one is immune to postpartum depression. I am one of so many women whose disorder was life-shattering, but I managed to get through the dark abyss, and I made it out to the other side—battered, broken, and bruised, but alive. The Centers for Disease Control and Prevention report that postpartum depression affects 10–15 percent of all mothers within the first year of giving birth. By some estimates, this means that there are over 950,000 cases of postpartum depression each year in the United States alone, and though this number is staggering, it is also presumably so much lower than the actual number of sufferers, as many cases go unreported, and many women ail in silence.[1]

Many people are familiar with the general notion of postpartum depression, but the afflictions of prenatal anxiety and prenatal depression, from which I also suffered, are not publicized, not understood and, therefore, all too often, not treated. Yet perinatal distress, which occurs both during and after pregnancy, affects so many women. Too many women.

I am one reported case. I have been able to shout out the things that many can only speak about in a whisper—that many cannot speak about at all. I am only here today because I had a husband who saw the light flicker and then extinguish from my eyes; I had a support system, fortified by my family members, closest friends, and an expert treatment team, who kept me safe from myself; I had access to medicine and hospitals. Like I said, I am one of the lucky ones. Many women are not so fortunate.

It could have panned out differently for me. In my darkest of days, I knew that I loved my children deeply, and I knew that I was grateful for their existence, but I could feel nothing but despair. At my worst, I just felt numbness. I could not feel anything at all. And though it may seem counterintuitive, I can tell you that when you can feel nothing, there is nothing more painful.

My children—my beautiful children, who radiate warmth, and goodness, and empathy, and resilience—could not prevent that abyss. However, with them, and because of them, I feel deeply, and I feel profoundly, and I often feel as though my heart could explode out of my chest with the love it holds inside. They shattered my numbness.

My daughter, Annabelle—our Belle—was born in April 2010. With Belle I had a clinically normal pregnancy, with a manageable amount of anxiety. She was (she is) my dream come true, and while pregnant with her, and after she was born, and today, I have worried about her safety and health and well-being. Before she was born, I did call the OBGYN with numerous questions ("I just drank expired ice tea! Will that cause permanent damage?" and "She usually kicks for, like, ten minutes after I eat chocolate, but this time she only kicked for, like, two minutes. Is she okay?" and "The restaurant I just went to accidentally served me tonic water instead of club soda! Does she have quinine poisoning? No? Well, what are the symptoms of quinine poisoning, just so that we can be sure?"). The doctor and nurse at my practice always served to assuage my fears ("You're fine!" and "Just sit with your feet up, and see what happens," and "You really, really are fine!").

Once Belle was born, I continued to worry about her safety and health and well-being, but at a level that was considered normal (statistically average) for a new mom. I was the first of my friends to have a baby, and I did not have a network of moms or any semblance of a mom village. I did not yet own an iPhone, therefore making the mastery of one-handed Googling while breastfeeding nearly impossible. Whereas today answers are at the tips of our fingers, in my early days with Belle I often felt as though we were on an island. A glittery, tutu-covered one, but an island nonetheless.

I know, now, that Belle's birth scared me and that this fear crept in, stealthily (perhaps through my cesarean-section opening), and then, while being ignored, silently infiltrated all of my cells, into my whole being. While in labor with Belle, I had to have an unplanned, eleventh-hour, rushed cesarean section and found out that her umbilical cord was wrapped around her neck twice. Immediately after she was born, instead of focusing on the scary birth experience I'd just endured, I had in my arms a tiny, beautiful human on which to dote and for whom to care. I had pink, tie-dyed onesies and headbands with giant flowers, and in the kaleidoscope of ruffles and sparkles, my view was obscured. I did not have a chance to deal with how my harrowing delivery had affected me and, as a result, as I now know, did not set myself up for future success. Where I could have developed fortitude, I only fostered fear. Because, while motherhood was hard, it was also enchanting.

With Belle I learned that when you are a mother, your heart, as they say, can often feel as though it is on the outside of your body. After she was born I had a case of the "baby blues," which for me meant that I was exhausted, nervous, and weepy, all normal symptoms for a mother within the first couple of weeks after giving birth.

I remember, so vividly, a visit to my parents' house when Belle was just a few weeks old. I had been holding it together, swallowing my feelings of angst, until the dam finally broke. As I sank into the large, leather armchair in their family room, I admitted to my mom that I was overwhelmed.

"I feel like I'm trapped in a hamster wheel and can't stop the spinning," I choked out, tears streaming down my cheeks.

She came over to me and put her arms around me, and she let me cry into her shoulder, without judgment or reproach—without even saying a word.

"You know those days when you have a million things scheduled, and you know that it's going to be a hard day, and so you dread it, but then you get through it and just breathe? I feel like that is *every day* for me, and I'm living one of those hard days, over and over, in three-hour cycles."

My mom explained to me that she had felt the same way when she was a new, young mother with me and that the newborn days are so hard and so draining, but she assured me that I would sleep again. I found so much solace in her validation. My mom carved out a space for me in which I could admit my darkest truths—which, at the time, were not all that dark. She did not just assuage my anxieties about chronic sleep-deprivation and exhaustion but, more than that, allayed my fears that my having these woes meant I was not a good mother. I felt heard. I know, too, that many women do not find that comfort in others.

Yes, I was tired, but I was also joyful, grateful, and madly in love. Life was colorful. We danced.

Three and a half years later, in October 2013, my Beau came into this world, and everything changed. From the moment I found out that I was pregnant with him, life shifted. I suffered from prenatal anxiety and depression, something that I did not even know existed until it swallowed me whole. I worried constantly, without reprieve; I was unable to connect with the baby growing inside of me; I could not even choose baby clothing for him, because when I would go shopping, all of the baby-boy clothing was covered in light blue and teddy bears, and during that time I hated anything with light blue and teddy bears.

For the first six weeks of my pregnancy, my anxious feelings were intense and inescapable. It was as if I were going through life without a layer of skin, so that anything—from the smallest gust of wind to the lightest touch—caused searing pain. I was terrified that something would go wrong, and I ruminated, endlessly, playing out all of the possible scary scenarios over and over in my head.

After a spotting-related scare when I was six weeks pregnant, I ended up in the emergency room. Hours later, emotionally wrecked from the trauma of the experience, I walked out of the hospital doors with two things: paperwork that read "possible miscarriage" and the sense of complete, utter, all-encompassing numbness. I was no longer scared; I no longer felt anything at all.

A little over seven months later, when Alexander Beau—our Beau—was born, I loved him instantly and fiercely. My numbness was replaced with a sense of euphoria, and I felt so relieved.

"I am back and better than ever," I thought to myself. I even *said* it to the people who were close to me: "I don't know what was wrong with me, but something about that pregnancy didn't agree with me. Now that he's here, I feel *amazing*."

I believed that the bad part—the crippling anxiety, the impending sense of doom, the cold emptiness—was behind me and that all I would carry from that moment forward would be my tiny baby, his big sister, and a feeling of contentment. I was so terribly, terrifyingly wrong.

Within a few days of my repeat cesarean section, I began to sink down into the dark place that I now know to be called severe postpartum depression. Whereas my postpartum experience with Belle had been hard, after having Beau I was debilitated. With Belle, even when I had felt utterly exhausted or wholly overwhelmed, I could still find joy and color in our lives. When I had Beau, all of the color just faded away. It was if I were on an eerie, gray-hued carousel I couldn't get off, and as I tried desperately to jump from horse to horse, each met me with a new worry or challenge or scary thought. In my worst moments, I lost the will to live.

After a month of suffering, spinning mercilessly in my own mind, I began to seek help. First, I used talk therapy with a psychiatrist and then, for the first time in my life, medication. I was put on several antidepressant medications: Prozac (a selective serotonin reuptake inhibitor, or, commonly, SSRI) and Wellbutrin (an aminoketone), as well as an anxiety medication (a benzodiazepine). Though this combination was helpful, it was still no match for my depression. I needed a higher level of care, including a mood-stabilizing medicine (Zyprexa, known as an atypical antipsychotic). I resisted this new drug, because at the time I had been informed that small amounts of the medication could pass from mother to baby when breastfeeding.[2] Ultimately, the choice was taken from me. In my darkest hour, when I saw nothing but bleakness, I was told that I needed to take the mood stabilizer "or else" and that I could no longer breastfeed my son. But breastfeeding was the one thing that still made me feel useful to him. I had failed him in every other way. After having breastfed Belle for eighteen months, losing the ability to nurse my baby Beau at ten weeks added a double shot of guilt to my constant cocktail of anxiety, depression, panic, and pain.

Almost immediately after I started to take the proper medication, something amazing happened: the medicine began to work. Color started to bloom back into view. The light started to return, slowly, to my eyes. I wanted to live once more. Though my existence did not feel enchanting, it felt worth living. I held my son, and I hugged my daughter, and I collapsed into my husband, and I knew that they all needed me, and I felt a sense of purpose once again. It was at that time that I heard an expression about breastfeeding that has stuck with me ever since: *It is better for your baby to have a mom without a boob than a boob without a mom.* My child would be better served by a healthy mother than by a plagued zombie shell of a human who could provide him with breast milk.

In the years following Beau's birth I have continued to live what I call my "hopeful story." I still see therapists, take medication, and have regular, predictable, free-floating anxiety. I also see bright colors, take my kids out for ice cream breakfast dates, and have daily dance parties. Together, as a family, we twirl around on our hardwood floors, using our slippery socks for momentum; the kids ask me to play them "like a guitar," which involves my holding Belle or Beau upside down and strumming on their stomachs as they giggle, uncontrollably; Kenny and I slow dance together, swaying our hips and locking our eyes, as our kids swing each other around by the arms, their laughter often drowning out the music. Even when life is not beautiful, we try to find the beauty in the small, in-between moments.

Don't get me wrong—not all of the in-between moments are lovely and picturesque. Motherhood is still messy, mercurial, hard, scary, stressful, lonely, boring, cluttered, and overwhelming. Yes, I adore my children, and, yes, they stress me out. As they have grown, so have their needs.

I have often described the experience of parenting Belle like this: Belle is the result of what would have happened if I, Becca, had been raised by myself, Becca, instead of by my own more even-keeled, perhaps reserved, quieter mother. Becca being mothered by Becca is like Becca times a million, and that makes Belle a force of nature. Her emotional needs are vast, her homework is now so challenging that even I, sometimes, need help when helping her with it, and she is the only human on Earth who talks as much as I do; my parents say that this is my ultimate payback. They say it with a smile, though, of course, as both she and I talk incessantly, but she and I also bring them tremendous joy, and they love us both so dearly. Our mouths just never stop running.

Parenting Beau is a completely different experience. So many of the things that I was scared of when I found out that I was having a boy (having grown up in a house with girls) are the things I love most. While we do not adhere to traditional gender stereotypes in our house, Beau has fully embraced all of the things that you would, let's say, find in the "boy aisle" of the toy store. He loves superheroes and Star Wars, the latter of which I had previously vowed to never see. I am scared of outer space. But he loves these things, which makes me love these things, and I recently found myself drawing an extensive family tree to explain the connections between the characters in the Star Wars universe (did you know that Darth Vader is Han Solo's father-in-law??). Beau is also extremely stubborn and smart as a whip, which is a glorious and challenging combination. His big brain just never stops running.

My house is always messier than I would like. The kids know how to push each other's buttons, and one will often try to surreptitiously antagonize the other over things as small as a rogue Rice Krispy. Despite my aversion to the sound of loud noises, they yell, even though they know they are not supposed to. Kenny yells, although he works hard not to. Belle and Beau will repeat their points, or requests, ad nauseum, and sometimes their refrain is expressed so loudly that it's hard to not acquiesce to their demands just to make the noise stop. Parenting is a juggling act, and I am constantly trying to simultaneously hold on to both virtue and survival.

There are some days when I feel like a good mom. The days when I have checked the boxes that my brain has arbitrarily created for me. The days when I have taken them to an activity and made them smile and given them a nutritious meal and introduced them to a new song.

There are days when I feel like a bad mom, and all of those unchecked boxes feel so heavy and burdensome and sit on my chest until I do something about them. The days when I keep Belle and Beau cooped up inside because I am tired or am short with them or have given them a crappy meal and they spend too much time watching television or playing video games. Oh, the guilt.

Then there are the quiet moments, when I feel the most like a mom— not a good mom or a bad mom, but simply, purely, the mommiest mom. The times when I wipe down the inside of a lunchbox and write a note to surprise Beau. The times when Belle asks me a hard, emotional question, and I tackle it, head on, and give her the truth, even when it is scary. When I sew up a hole in Beau's precious stuffy, Michael Woody, and he says, "Thank you for mending him." When Belle and I are up before anyone else in the house and sip hot cocoa together, pointing out the rainbow prisms on the walls, as the sun starts to peek in through the windows.

These days, when I'm happy, I feel that joy in every part of my body; I am living so deliberately and with gratitude. When I am sad, I cry, but I do not feel hopeless, and the future does not seem bleak. I feel emotions in a way that is clinically average and statistically normal. Today I am no longer the woman I was before my experience with severe perinatal anxiety and depression, but in most ways that is a good thing. When I had to climb my way back up from the bottom, it gave me strength in places I didn't know I had; my hands are now strong and capable from having clawed myself up out of my pit of despair; my legs are now more sturdy, serving as a solid foundation upon which the rest of me is grounded; my heart now beats in a new way, having been torn out, put back in, and repaired, and it continues to heal. After all, it's what keeps me alive.

I shared my story, of suffering and recovery, in real time, on the "mommy blog" I had started as my online baby book when Belle was just two months old. The blog grew, and more and more people across the world reached out to me to tell me that my story was their story, that their story was my story, that they could have written the same words I had just used, that they could finally feel less alone—that I was not alone. I started to repeat that message to others.

I wrote a book.

I have spoken all across the country about my story and my experience. I stood in front of the majestic US Capitol at the 2018 March for Moms and advocated for maternal mental health. I was deemed a VIP along with some of the nation's leading experts in health care, government officials, policy makers, television personalities, and influencers, like Christy Turlington, one of the most famous supermodels of all time. These people became my friends. We were all fighting the same fight, and nothing else mattered.

I spoke from atop the iconic steps of the Philadelphia Museum of Art and told the crowd at the 2019 Women's March that "it's okay to not be okay." I was among a group of esteemed politicians, like the state's attorney general and the city's mayor and controller. When I stepped up to the podium on that frigid January day, I looked out at the sea of supporters and said, "Five years ago, I never thought that I would be here, today," and I meant it in more ways than they could understand.

In one magazine interview I tried to describe the difference between the "baby blues" and true postpartum depression. First, I gave the clinical answer that had been taught to me by a therapist at the local postpartum-stress center. She said that baby blues are the negative emotions that we feel during the two weeks after giving birth. She said that any form of distress (like anxiety or depression) that begins or persists after the first two weeks falls somewhere on the spectrum of postpartum depression.

But then I gave the interviewer my own definition. I talked about being able to find joy and then not, about color versus gray. It was then that I said something that had been on the tip of my tongue for the five years since my Beau had been born but had never quite been able to articulate or even access.

"Belle is the child that I always dreamed of having," I said. "She is the living embodiment of my dreams having come true, and she allowed me to be the mother I had always dreamed of being. Beau is the child I had never expected. He is more incredible than I could have ever imagined, and he has allowed me to be the mother I could have never imagined but who I was meant to be."

In these five years, I have not returned to the person I was before my experience with severe perinatal distress; rather, I have become someone new. I have grown up. I have found my voice.

But despite all of my growth and strength and progress, and despite the joy I feel in my heart that literally feels like the warmth in my chest is radiating through my entire body, I also feel something else. Something less lovely and strong and healed and right. I feel a hole. This hole has been with me for the past five years, and no matter what I have done to try and close it, it continues to find its way open. Unlike Michael Woody, this hole is one that I do not know how to mend. The hole, I now realize, is in the shape of a baby.

Because I had almost lost my life when suffering from severe postpartum depression, I was told at twenty-eight years old that I should no longer have children, as doing so would likely put my life in jeopardy. This is a part of my story that is hard to discuss for many different reasons.

On one hand, the feelings of grief and loss I experience after being told to not have another child make me feel guilty, as I already have two children, a girl and a boy, and I feel so fortunate for them, every minute of every day. Even when I am not enjoying motherhood, I am appreciating motherhood. I am grateful in a way that I will never be able to describe. I carried these babies in my own body. I was able to feel them move inside of me, first like tiny butterfly wings fluttering, and then as big kicks, like little earthquakes shaking me from the inside out. I delivered both of these babies via cesarean-section surgeries, and while I did not particularly enjoy my birth experiences, I was there to hear them each cry, with loud, strong, staccato wails in the operating rooms. I was able to hear the nurses call out, "Seven pounds, twelve ounces," for each of my babies—as they were both born at the exact same size. I nursed these babies, I held them and rocked them and changed them and snuggled them. I know how much it means to welcome a baby. I know that there are so many people who would do anything to be in my position of having two healthy children, and that makes it hard for me to admit to wanting more. It makes me feel greedy and ungrateful, and perhaps it makes me seem like I don't fully appreciate my good fortune; perhaps it makes it seem that I am unappreciative of all that I have. But life is not a zero-sum game. For me—just like for any woman who longs for a child and to be a mother because somewhere inside she feels incomplete—I feel an uncomfortable emptiness.

I can no longer have children.

On the other hand—the hand of mine that trembles as it types and the hand that wipes the tears that form in my eyes—it is hard to write about not having more children because it makes me feel so very sad. Despite the gratitude I feel for my children, the baby-shaped hole in my heart makes me feel both lost and like I *have* lost.

One night, as I was under my covers, listening to a podcast, trying to fall asleep, I heard something so interesting that I shot up from my bed, replayed it, and wrote it down. It was further support for a belief that I had been employing, and sharing, about dialectical reasoning. Bret Weinstein, a notable biologist and evolutionary theorist, was being interviewed on *Armchair Expert*, a podcast hosted by Dax Shepard, a notable actor and comedian. During his interview, Weinstein said, "One of the keys to human uniqueness is the fact that we can literally hold two views that cannot be reconciled simultaneously and have what amounts to a literal argument with ourselves about the truth of it. And the ability to do that puts us in a great position to discover what we don't know—basically, to bootstrap knowledge."[3]

I can use dialectical thinking, and I can intellectualize the situation, and I can try to move through the stages of grief, but the hole remains. After hearing the aforementioned interview, I took to Twitter, a social media platform that I seldom use, and sent a thank-you to both Bret Weinstein and Dax Shepard. They both replied—Dax with a series of smiley-face and heart emojis, Bret with this: "It's early days for the integration of evolutionary thinking into mental health fields, but nothing could be more important."[4] I felt so validated.

At such a young age (at least by today's standards) I was told that it would no longer be safe for me to have more children, as my body and brain would likely turn against me, and no matter how unfair this felt (feels), it also informed how my husband, parents, and loved ones were able to process my grief. To them, having the option of a future pregnancy taken off the table was a relief. To them, it was a way to safeguard me from myself, as they were the ones who had also been to hell when I had grown so sick. They were the ones who had to pick me up off of the floor, and break down the doors, and pull the razor blades out of my hands and remove all of the sharp objects from my house to prevent me from continuing to engage in my self-harming behaviors.

When I try to empathize with my family members, and imagine how they must feel, I can so keenly understand their positions, both intellectually and emotionally.

I think back to one dark, winter night when Beau was just a couple of months old and my parents brought both kids to their home for a special date. Kenny had taken a rare moment to sit and just zone out in front of the television in our sunroom. I had taken that rare opportunity to sneak upstairs and into the hall bathroom, close the door behind me, and disassemble a disposable razor that had been left behind after the most obvious hazards (Kenny's razor blades, our kitchen knives) had already been removed during the first sweep of our house. I'd found the razor and used a pair of tweezers to pull it apart and dragged the blade across the top of my left forearm. My arm was already mangled, with lines in different stages of hurting and healing, like a sunset, the colors ranging from tan to pink to angry red. It was what a sunset might look like in hell. When Kenny realized that I'd been gone for too long, he came up to find I had locked myself in the bathroom. He kicked down the door and pulled the blade from the trembling hand that was attached to my bleeding arm.

And that was not the only such traumatic night, nor was it the worst night. There was so much darkness and devastation during that period. One time, so desperate to hurt myself, I had climbed up on the kitchen counter in order to access the highest shelf, above the stove. I rummaged through the thick, cherrywood encasement until I found what I was looking for: our mandolin, still in its packaging, its blades still so sharp they were as slick as ice. My family members found me that time before I could hurt myself. That was a bad time.

Anything that could possibly prevent me from going back to that dark place again seemed like a very good thing to everyone who loves me.

But it has never felt good to me. And this is a complicated notion to reconcile. I know that, because I have suffered from severe prenatal and postpartum anxiety and depression, I am now at a much greater risk for suffering from these afflictions again. I know that a previous bout with prenatal or postpartum depression is one of the biggest risk factors for developing the same afflictions in a future pregnancy. I survived last time—both physically and emotionally—but it was brutal. And I am responsible for two children who need me. In many ways, my longing for another child feels selfish. But admitting it is also honest.

For me, the world is filled with land mines. I am surrounded by pregnancy announcements and belly bumps and tiny, cute, swaddled bundles of baby. Every time I log on to social media, I am hit with a tiny-moccasin-style announcement (or two). When I check the news for pertinent current-events updates, I'm bombarded with what are now commonly referred to as "bumpdates." I am supremely happy for the people announcing their pregnancies or the births of their children, but at the same time, some of the time, it hurts. The most painful, for me, is when it is the announcement of a third child. It is something so specific that I want so badly and may never have. I look at these announcements, and, as embarrassing as it is for me to admit, I covet what they have. The emptiness I carry grows even deeper; the hole is more gaping. Like I said, I can tell you that there is nothing more painful than when you can feel nothing.

I have gotten used to the questions and the answers that surround me as a woman of childbearing age.

The questions come from everyone, everywhere. People ask whether I am done having children. They ask whether my children want a sibling. When I am in a medical situation, especially when I am being given a new medicine or scheduling a procedure, I am asked whether I could be pregnant or plan to try to get pregnant in the near future. In the hardest of situations, I am forced to take a "standard" pregnancy test to confirm that I am definitely, positively, 100 percent not pregnant. And that definitely, positively, 100 percent feels like a hammer to my sometimes-fragile heart.

Quite often people do not even ask me a question, but rather they give me their unsolicited opinions and "answers." They tell me that I am so lucky to have what I have. They tell me that I am certainly done because I have a girl and a boy, as if that is the only ideal imaginable. They tell me, "With two children, you and your husband get to parent with man-to-man coverage, but when you add a third, then you have to go to zone defense." In my head, I tell them to mind their own business, to keep their hands off of my playbook, or something less polite. Why shouldn't I be allowed to want, and pursue, the family that I had envisioned? Some people want one child, some want ten. Shouldn't we all be able to try for the things we want? To form the families that we create and dream of and hold in our hearts—often before we can do so in our arms?

I know all of the questions, and I know all of the answers. But there is the rational brain, and then there is the emotional brain. The emotional part of me is where the hole lives, all cute baby-shaped and warm and good smelling and magical. There is a part of me that believes, in the core of my being, that there is this little baby out there, waiting for me, whom I will never know. That this baby should exist. And that I'm missing it.

I picture this absence in all different ways, but one image I always find myself returning to is of a giant, fortress-like castle. It is guarded and, on all sides, surrounded by water. There is a baby on one side of the moat, and me, helpless, on the other. The baby is calling out to me, begging me to find a way across the water. I try to leap, and I fall. I start to build a bridge, and it collapses. I decide to brave the water, and I'm met with alligators or dragons or other unknown creatures who will not let me pass—who will not let me get to the other side.

"Please, Mommy! Please find me!" cries the baby.

"I'm trying, Baby!" I scream across the water. "I see you! I'm trying to get you! Mommy is trying!"

Mommy.

Baby.

It breaks my heart.

The shop is closed, they say. And so I live my life appreciating all that I have, enjoying these new, fun stages of my children's lives, and tucking the pain away.

I stare into Belle's face, her big eyes rimmed by a leathery whip of black lashes, her lips the exact shape of my own, full and with points like an arrow, and I swell with pride for the little lady she has become. She astounds me with her compassion, awes me with her way with words, and takes my breath away with her beauty.

I feel so lucky to be her mom.

I stare into Beau's eyes, bright blue and crystalline like glowing marbles, his hair thick and strawberry blond, never ceasing to surprise me, and I say a silent thank-you to him for allowing me to become the person I am today. He amazes me with his strength, impresses me with his tenacity, and makes me well up with tears over his quiet sensitivity.

I feel so lucky to be his mom.

When Beau was first born, I remember writing a caption on a photo of the two of them: "Team Starr, Est. 2013," it read, under a picture of baby Beau clutching little Belle's hand. To say that they are a team would be an understatement. They are the best of friends and have created an enchanted world of their own, like a snow globe—with a beautiful scene inside, but encased, preciously, within a bubble—and while I can see it, I cannot really enter it; I am a mere spectator. They have code words and inside jokes and original songs, and they make each other laugh in a way that spreads the joy in their giggles to everyone around them. When they bring out the best in each other, they applaud one another's successes. When they are naughty and break a rule or two, they cover for each other. They belong to each other.

I have two extraordinary children who are evolving into extraordinary humans. They both have a preternatural level of empathy that transcends age or size or time.

They finally have a mother who is present and stable and well.

But then, each day as I wake and each night as I rest my head and in a thousand moments in between, I see the baby from across the moat, and I hear its cries, and the hole in my heart aches, so deeply, that it can bring me to my knees.

"I'm trying, Baby," I whisper to myself, not sure who I am trying to reassure.

I am trying. I'm not sure what I'm trying, but I am trying. Trying to heal. Trying to close the hole. Trying not to hope. Trying to find peace.

And at the same time still trying to figure out a way to get safely across the moat.

2

❖ ❖

Or Is It?

In April 2017, life decided to, once again, do a pirouette. We were out from under the blazing forest fire that was acute postpartum depression. Gray smoke was no longer billowing from the sky, undulating, daily, toward our family, threatening to swallow us whole in its darkness. But we could still smell the smoke. No matter how hard we scrubbed ourselves clean, the scent lingered. No matter how many times I dusted, when I ran my finger over any surface of our home, I would still find traces of soot. And, frankly, I did not have the energy to keep scrubbing or dusting over and over and over again. Our family was healing, *I was healing*, and we watched, with gratitude and awe, as our sky went from black to gray to orange to pink to white to blue.

While life was colorful, again, it was also mercurial. We were in a dance, and while one foot remained on the ground, everything else began to spin. In March 2017, just one month prior, my mother-in-law had suffered a bad fall and been taken to the hospital, and it had soon become apparent that she was finally beginning to succumb to her nineteen-year battle with Parkinson's disease. I had never known Susan, Kenny's mom, when she was not sick, but the disease had progressed profoundly throughout my nearly twelve years with her. Her Parkinson's disease impacted her mobility, and by the time she fell on that bitterly cold March morning, she had already been using a wheelchair or scooter almost full time. After her fall, she slipped into a disoriented state of progressive dementia, and, for her safety and well-being, we moved her to a skilled rehab and memory-care nursing facility. Kenny had also just lost his father a year and a half prior, and after having only just been able to take off his caretaker uniform from his struggles with my depression, he had to don another caretaker suit once again, albeit of a different sort, for his mom.

It was a very weird time in our lives.

It was a chilly morning at the end of April 2017 when I had to face my own medical scare. Since Belle's birth, and subsequent eighteen months of breastfeeding, I had been monitored for a benign mass of extra breast tissue between the outer edge of my right breast and right axillary area. Read: side boob.

Incidentally, I had also discovered some other palpable lymph nodes, both under that arm and along my groin. I called the Hospital of the University of Pennsylvania and described my symptoms to the coordinator, who told me that she would relay my information to HUP's breast and surgical oncology teams and would get back to me with their feedback. While I waited, anxiously, for her call, I dressed myself for an afternoon tea date. Obviously.

I had made plans to have proper tea out in the western suburbs of Philadelphia with a sweet friend. My friend, by nature, is elegant and sophisticated, and afternoon tea, by nature, feels elegant and sophisticated, and so I tried to look the part. I traded my studded Jimmy Choo moto boots for the black Chanel ballet flats I had gotten for my twenty-second birthday. I pulled my hair back into a neat chignon and, as I often did in those days—a time when so much felt uncertain—wore a piece belonging to my mother-in-law, in this case a silk scarf, wrapped loosely around my neck and knotted in the center. *Literally* fancy pants.

As my friend and I sat with our delicate mugs of tea, array of tiny sandwiches, and deluge of stories pouring from our lips, I got a call from a Philadelphia number.

I answered with both eagerness and trepidation.

"Rebecca?" the kind hospital coordinator began. "The oncology team and the breast surgeons want to see you. But there's a catch. They need to see you now. They can only see you if you get here by 2 P.M. Can you make it?"

I looked down at the plate before me, with my half-eaten egg salad and cucumber sandwiches, and then at the time. It was 1:40. To put this in perspective, I live right outside of Philadelphia proper, in the suburban town that is three train stops away from being across City Line. For afternoon tea I had driven away from the city, an additional ten train stops further from where I would need to meet the medical team, which was at the hospital in West Philadelphia.

Feeling frenzied, I apologized to my friend, got up from the table, and headed east on Route 30, a main road running through Philadelphia's storied Main Line suburb. I was frazzled by so many things at once—leaving my friend in such a rude and jarring manner, the intense pressure to make it down to the hospital on time, the knowledge that a team of oncological surgeons had been told about my symptoms and wanted to see me as quickly as possible, the fact that it was a few days before my next waxing appointment. Out of all of the things to focus on, and perhaps as a coping mechanism of sorts, I felt a desperate urge to be able to shave my legs and bikini line before they were examined by the surgeons at the hospital. I was on the phone with my mom, telling her about what I had been instructed to do, planning with her where we would meet (because, of course, the moment I told my mom that the oncologists wanted to see me, she left work in Center City Philadelphia to come meet me at the hospital), and stopped to say, "Hold on—I have to run into this Rite Aid."

I will confess that I am someone who prides herself on always having shaved legs. This is 40 percent fueled by a combination of feeling good about myself and also feeling like I have not "let myself go" after over a decade of marriage and 60 percent fueled by fear of winding up in the exact situation I found myself in. Every time I am in the shower, I think, "Just take the extra two minutes to shave. Let's say you end up in the emergency room today."

I wish I were kidding.

My mom told me to keep driving, that I was being ridiculous, and the quickest way to get to the area of the hospital where I needed to be. I jerked my car abruptly into the left lane and then made a sharp left into the parking lot of the big, blue drug store, where I raced toward the disposable-razor aisle.

It was a measure of self-preservation, I think. I would not be able to control anything that was about to happen to me, but I could absolutely make sure that, whatever happened, I would handle it with very smooth legs.

By some miracle, I got to the hospital on time, met my mom, threw my keys at the man in charge of the valet-parking service, pushed my way into the revolving, glass door—awkwardly, so that I was one of those people who chose to share the little compartment with another person—held hands with my mom as we squeezed into a packed elevator, and rode up to the oncology floor. The oncology floor is a terrifying place to be.

I managed my anxiety by finding the closest private bathroom, pulling down my pants, hovering over the sink, wrestling with some very inconvenient plastic packaging, breaking out my new razor, and shaving. I was about to be examined for palpable, suspicious lymph nodes in multiple areas of my body—on the very same hospital floor where several members of my family had been given bad, malignant diagnoses—and I was using the time to contort my body so that I would not get razor burn as I shaved, using lukewarm hospital water and foamy hospital soap and rough hospital paper towels. It was so weird.

My mom interrupted me by knocking on the bathroom door and telling me that it was our turn to be seen. I was met by a young male surgeon who asked me to lie down on the exam table so he could palpate my lymph-nodey groin. I silently thanked myself for having insisted on the Rite Aid detour. He told me that the nodes, while present, felt normal to him. I told him that they did not feel normal to me; they felt cancery. He explained that because of my low weight and lack of body fat, everything would feel more prominent on my body. I gave him my best "But these really do feel cancery to me" face. He sent me for an ultrasound.

The next step on my journey was down to the ground floor, where I would get a mammogram, breast ultrasound, and the aforementioned groin ultrasound and meet with a different surgeon. In the radiology area, I was told that I had to strip down to just a hospital gown and shoes. For the next few hours I found myself walking around with nothing but baby-soft legs, an XL snap-on hospital gown, and my Chanel ballet flats.

"Only *me*," I said to myself.

But, remarkably, this wasn't the first time I'd found myself so attired in a hospital. Just to add a little color commentary to this story, I will share this side note, which also serves to explain some of my hypochondriac tendencies. Three years earlier, after a burst pipe had caused a massive flood in our basement, our home's old boiler had malfunctioned, causing it to emit carbon monoxide. We did not know this initially, of course, but I had started to feel lightheaded that night before retiring to bed. Thinking I might be suffering from low blood sugar, I ate a late-night Luna Bar, drank some water, and went to sleep, only to be woken up at five in the morning to the sound of the carbon-monoxide detector blaring. We called 911, and the moment the fire department crew showed up and took a reading, their hand-held detector started to blare even more shrilly than our still-beeping in-home alarm. I had to rush outside in nothing but my pajama pants and a thin, white tank. Because I was symptomatic, I was taken to the local hospital with bare feet and unquantifiable amount of gratitude. When my husband arrived at the hospital with our two kids—both of whom also had carbon monoxide in their blood—he handed me the first pair of my shoes he'd been able to grab out of our closet before rushing out the door: my Chanel ballet flats.

And so, finding myself, once again, near-naked in a hospital, wearing nothing but a thin gown and those designer shoes, I had to laugh. While we sat in the sterile waiting room at HUP, my mom and I noted the complete ridiculousness in the situation. It was so preposterous that it was funny— that is, if anything can, in any way, be funny while shared when sitting in the radiology unit of a hospital, awaiting a mammogram and consult with an oncological surgeon.

It was in the HUP radiology unit that I reunited with my husband again, as he, like my mom, had raced to be by my side. My mammogram came back with a normal reading, and after the physician did an ultrasound on my right axillary area, she told me that my breasts "looked beautiful."

"Well, that is the first time I have heard *that* in years," I said, half-laughing, awkwardly.

I was then sent to a different area of the unit, where a male technician would be looking at the nodes in my groin. He was so kind, and though, as a technician, he was not supposed to say anything diagnostic, he was willing to assuage some of my anxieties in ways that other techs in the past had not. While in that final exam room, my mind was brought back to my traumatic emergency-room visit when I was newly pregnant with Beau. It had been Saint Patrick's Day evening, I was six weeks pregnant, and I had started spotting. Already feeling intense prenatal anxiety, this episode threw me. While that ultrasound technician was giving me a transvaginal exam, she had kept the monitor turned away from me and remained stone-faced for the entire examination as she probed me from the inside. When I asked her whether the baby inside of me was okay—whether there even *was* a baby inside of me—she refused to answer, explaining that the doctor would give me a full report after consulting with the radiologist. In the hours between that ultrasound and my visit from the emergency-room attending doctor, I was left alone with my increasingly scary thoughts. I worried for the baby I had yet to see, I worried for Belle and how we would explain a possible loss, and I worried for myself and what it would feel like if all of the worries I had been feeling proved to be correct. Of course, they were not, and the baby, then shaped like a tiny Cheerio, had a strong heartbeat and later turned into my Beau.

And so four years later, as I stretched out on the table for a very different kind of ultrasound, the kind technician ran his wand across my pelvis. He kept the monitor facing me, and although I did not know quite what to look out for, I joked to Kenny and my mom about how decidedly less exciting this was than any other ultrasound I could remember. No flickering grain of rice; no Cheerio; no peeking between tiny, barely distinguishable legs; no baby.

As he continued to examine my right side, the gentle technician told me that everything looked really good, and while he could feel the lymph nodes along my bikini line, they did not have malignant qualities. Then he said that he would be taking a look my ovaries.

When he pressed down, I did not feel anything.

"I guess I am not ovulating from that side this month," I said, casually. I like to keep things casual when people are wielding tools around my groin area.

As soon as he pressed down on the left side, I winced at the tenderness.

"Yup. That's where I'm ovulating," I told him, flatly.

"Wow, you know your body well! Look at this giant follicle you have here. Look at all of these eggs!"

I felt a flash of pain jolt me from somewhere deep inside.

"What a waste," I thought to myself, feeling a surge of anger for my own fertility.

Kenny, still sitting next to me, saw the tears forming in my eyes. He reached out and held my hand. He knew why this was so hard for me—torturous, really. Even though it was irrational, to me each of those swaying grapes on the monitor represented the loss of something—someone—whom I would never know. The loss of the promise of a possible someone to come.

"It's just so unfair," I lamented to Kenny, holding back my tears, as the tech continued to examine the suspicious lymph nodes in my groin. "I didn't ask for this to happen to me. I didn't ask for postpartum depression. And I have all of these eggs, and I know when I am ovulating, and it doesn't matter anymore. I just wish I had another chance. I wish we could try again."

The pain in my chest was crushing. I wanted another baby—and had never stopped wanting another baby—but I had been benched, permanently, because I had suffered from severe prenatal and postpartum depression three years prior.

Kenny looked at me, then back at the screen, then back at me, staring straight into my eyes.

"Maybe we can," he said, squeezing my hand a bit harder.

And then all of the tears I had been holding back flooded from my eyes, soaking my face and then the thin cotton hospital gown.

Maybe we can.

Postpartum depression leaves a lot of collateral damage. Some is to be expected, like the disruption to a couple's marriage among other traumas to unpack in one's family. People who have suffered from severe postpartum depression, like I did, are forever labeled: they (we) do not just have a preexisting condition; they (we) *are* a preexisting condition. We are fragile, vulnerable, and, perhaps damaged yet at the same time should feel grateful for having survived; we are stronger than ever—warriors.

But there is another, silent casualty to postpartum depression, and it is one that I did not see coming until I tripped over a camouflaged piece of shrapnel and it cut me at my knees. I cannot speak for everyone (though this has been a consistent theme in all of the conversations I have had with fellow survivors), and so I will only speak for myself when I say that people in my life are not nearly as supportive of future family expansion because I now have a history of having suffered from postpartum depression. This is more painful than I can convey.

Years prior, when the time had come for me to consider having a second child, my family members and friends had been encouraging, supportive, excited and even, in some cases, insistent. When I had told my dad that I was pregnant with my second child, presenting him with a pee stick with two lines on it, displayed on my fireplace mantel, he hugged me, beaming. When I had called my mom to tell her over the phone, she got teary-eyed. When I had FaceTimed my sister in New York, she jumped up and down. They all had been filled with joy and excitement. Like me, they were brimming with promise and hope. They'd had no reason *not* to be. I had done this before. It had gone so well. We had our Belle.

Pregnancy, for me, had, to that point, been healthy and glowy and enchanting.

And then everything changed. My next pregnancy sucked the life out of me. My loved ones watched me, helplessly, as I withered away into a hollow, gray shell. And because things had gotten so dark back then, the view today is still, so often, obscured. Even though I managed to turn things around and, once again, wanted to live, the only thing that anyone close to me can remember is the pain.

There is no one whom this impacts more acutely than Kenny.

When I'd first told him that I was pregnant with our second child, it had been warm and lovely. I had given Belle a small, rectangular box to hand to him, and when he opened it, he saw the positive pregnancy test. He'd smiled at me, and I'd smiled at him, and we were a team.

"Oh my God," we'd said. "We are going to have two kids."

I remember what I was wearing that day. It was a very soft pink-and-white-striped shirt with thumbholes that Kenny had given to me for Valentine's Day just a couple of weeks prior. Right after telling him the big news, our little family of three bundled up and went to the local library. We walked around the children's section, in the basement of the tiny building, and the two of us caught each other's eyes, over and over, and smiled. In those smiles we said,

"I can't believe this!"

and

"What have we gotten ourselves into?"

and

"This is amazing!"

and

"Belle is going to be a sister!"

and

"I love you."

It had all been so exciting and special and hopeful. Until it wasn't.

In my pursuit to have a third child, the baby that has been calling out for me for so long that I cannot remember a time when the hole did not exist in me, I have not been met with excitement. There has been no enthusiasm. Nothing has been glowy. There has been no enchantment.

People are skeptical, anxious, adamant, incredulous, confused, scared.

In so many ways, I know that I cannot blame them.

Since having my Beau, and since having suffered from severe prenatal and postpartum anxiety and depression, I have had to accept (succumb to?) the reality that those words—those facts—are often the ones that define my reality. I am so many things, both at different times and, also, at the same time, but no matter what hat I don in the moment, I am *always* a survivor. Though it is better than the alternative, of course, it is also a label that, sometimes, I would like to take off. Or at the very least I would like to have the option of doing so. Like when I am signing up for life insurance. Like when I am onstage, singing, in front of a crowd of rock and roll lovers. Like when I want to have another baby.

I think back to the time when I was at my worst, at the end of 2013 and the beginning of 2014, and I recognize that, then, I was a real danger to myself. I was engaging in self-harming behaviors—for the first and only time in my life. Today, I reconcile this horrific time by believing, with my whole heart, that it was not I who ran the sharp objects along my arm, but rather the demon who had taken me over. While I know I am the same human in a literal sense, in so many other ways, both palpable and profound, I am not. I do not even know the person who lived in my body during those months of agony.

There is one memory from that time that I consider the worst of all. I sat on the living room couch next to Kenny and asked him—no, pleaded with him—to let me die. I needed his blessing. He would not oblige, and he and my family then worked together and fought harder for me than ever. I made it. It was by the skin of my teeth, but I made it to the other side. To the hopeful story.

But before hope, more practical steps needed to be taken—or, more accurately, desperate attempts were necessary to gain control of a rogue ship blown from its mooring. In one particularly powerful turn of the wheel, Kenny decided we could never have any more children and got (what we now refer to as) a hasty vasectomy. He got snipped with little fanfare and no sperm saved. It did not matter; nothing would ever make him book a return ticket to the hell he had so narrowly escaped.

So of course I understand why my family members would be scared for me to go through another pregnancy and postpartum period. Despite my own confidence in myself and my team, it was my family members who had served on the front lines of this blustery maritime war. And they are still scarred. I feel for them, deeply.

But even knowing all of this, it is so hard, now, to go through this internal struggle without them. It is so hard to get behind a decision when everyone else in my life is on the other side. It is like a tug-of-war, with a rope tied in ornate sailor's knots, and I have been so strong and have dug my heels into the sand below my feet, and I have held on to this rough, worn, fraying rope for so long that my hands, once callused, have begun to bleed. And I stand here, and I pull for this baby, every single day, but I do so alone. On the other end of the rope, standing across from me, are the people whom I love and respect and *need* most. They are not trying to take something away from me; they are trying to keep me safe, in the only way they know how. But in pulling on the rope against me, they are hurting me more than they realize. They just can't stop. And so neither can I.

And with Kenny's three words in the hospital that day, I felt like, perhaps, I had someone else behind me, to help me and to pull on my side of the rope. The most important person of all.

Maybe we can.

I did not know what the path ahead would look like, but I knew that, after all of the suffering and all of the pain, it could, finally, lead me to my baby. And no matter the obstacles, I would fight like a mother to get there.

Part II

A HOPEFUL STORY

How does one have a baby after severe prenatal and postpartum anxiety and depression?

It is a valid question, as there is such limited data on the subject.

This question often follows the more popular question of "Why?" and it is still, mostly, unasked.

The topic of pregnancy after severe perinatal distress is a difficult one to tackle, and so most people do not. But we are fortunate to have some (albeit limited) literature on both therapeutic and medicinal studies on pregnant women who are at risk for perinatal mood disorders and treated before, during, and after pregnancy in order to combat these afflictions.

The chasm of the topic of family expansion after postpartum depression looks like a mere crack in the sidewalk compared to the large crevasse in the data around the topics of adoption and surrogacy after postpartum depression. Besides anecdotal work, I was unable to find anything legitimate on these topics, save some old threads on online message boards and forums. To me, that is not good enough. We deserve better.

It is here that I will be sharing data with you and all of the information I found during my deep dive into this topic. I will be sharing my own story here, and it is honest and volatile and intense and warm and real. I will also be presenting you with clinical data from medical doctors, researchers, psychologists, psychiatrists, and professionals in the perinatal field. In addition, I have the honor of sharing other women's stories with you; in many cases, these women have so beautifully and bravely written their own stories to be included in this text in an effort to help others.

However, as this is an honest exploration of the choices that are offered to us so we can expand our families after postpartum depression, you will find that it is not always an easy exploration, nor is it at all balanced. I do not—because I cannot—share an equal amount of data on pregnancy after postpartum depression (a topic that comparatively has been studied much more thoroughly) and surrogacy after postpartum depression (something so rarely mentioned in literature—or anywhere—that it is much more difficult to provide a fully comprehensive picture of the experience).

But this lack of data on surrogacy in itself is noteworthy. Most women who have suffered from postpartum depression and who wish to expand their families subsequently make the choice to do so by choosing to carry another baby themselves; this is the most popular way any family expands, and so it makes sense intuitively that more data would exist surrounding this topic, although choosing to carry a baby after postpartum depression is, of course, a more nuanced situation. Far fewer women expand their families after postpartum depression through adoption or surrogacy. Many, whom I respect deeply, decide not to have any more children, and it is important for those on this path to understand why this is not only a valid choice but also, in many cases, the wise choice.

Most important, we have choices. We are warriors, and we are brave, and that means we deserve the chance to choose how we confront the challenge. And we no longer have to do it alone.

3

Grand Reopening

The bathroom in the delivery room was large and sterile. The light blue-green shade of the tiles seemed to match the thin, worn fabric of my gown.

I looked into Linda's eyes and thanked her, over and over, for being there for me.

"Tell me again," I pleaded with her. "Do you promise you will be here for the whole delivery, no matter how long it takes?"

Linda had been my rock before, and I needed her; in that moment, it felt like I needed Linda more than anyone.

"I promise you I am not going anywhere, sweetie," she said. "I am here for the next four days anyway."

A wave of relief flooded me as I made my way over to the toilet, as Linda had instructed me to try to pee so that they could monitor my level of hydration. If I were well hydrated, Linda explained, she, as my nurse, could persuade the doctors to allow me to try for a vaginal birth after cesarean (VBAC). I looked down at the floor, and those pallid-looking tiles, to see the trail of water that had come trickling out from beneath my gown. It was my amniotic fluid, and in it I could see the sick-looking yellow-brown-green substance that I knew to be meconium.

"This looks just like when I had Belle," I said to myself—or to Linda. I cannot remember.

Meconium, for lack of a better description, is the baby's poop inside of the womb. Oftentimes meconium in the amniotic fluid is a sign of potential fetal distress and an indicator that delivery should happen as quickly as possible. When I had Belle, it was the presence of meconium when my water broke (read: burst, after days of trickling, when the on-call doctor stuck her hand as far into me as she could reach, in order to try to place a fetal heart monitor on Belle's head) that led to my unplanned cesarean section.

The familiar sight of meconium did not seem to ramp up my anxiety, as the anxiety had already been constant and consuming. I thought about what my doctor had told me when we had met to discuss this possible pregnancy—that, because of my prior surgeries, he might have to make new incisions, both internally and externally, instead of the more traditional approach of going back through the scars from the old cesarean sections.

Linda had torn perfect squares from the toilet-paper holder mounted to the wall, and she lined the toilet seat for me, as if the hygiene in my hospital room were a top priority. Between my unwieldy body and my nervous shaking, I kept knocking the paper off the toilet seat, and she kept having to reline the seat for me, each time with the perfectly shaped squares. The floor was covered with toilet paper and meconium and amniotic fluid and tears.

"Just sit down, sweetie, and try to pee." She looked at me with her kind, light-colored eyes; her short, dirty-blonde hair was tucked just behind her ears.

It was the moment of truth. My pee would seal my fate in terms of this delivery, and I had tremendous performance anxiety, so to speak. I am always someone with some pee-related stage fright, but with the gravity of the moment I could not get my pelvic muscles to relax, and when Linda heard liquid drop into the toilet water, I had to confess to her that it was just my leaking sac and not urine.

Finally, after what seemed like an eternity, I was able to relax my muscles and release, and just as it was time to look into the toilet bowl to see whether I would be able to try to deliver this baby without surgery, I felt a hand shoving my shoulder, lightly.

"Mommy?" said a small, husky voice.

It was Beau, with his signature morning hoarseness.

"Mommy? Can I wake up Daddy?"

Confused, with my eyes closed, I wondered how Beau had gotten into the delivery room—and why Kenny was asleep during this pivotal moment.

I opened my eyes to see two bright blue eyes staring at me, my son's face so close to mine that I could feel his breath on my cheeks.

Had I been dreaming?

Yes.

I had been dreaming.

"But it felt so real," I said aloud.

Beau continued to hound me, but I was lost in my thoughts, with one foot still stuck in my dream, not wanting to let go. Linda was no longer by my side; Linda does not exist. In the light of day, the Linda in my dream most resembles a nurse named Joy, who had helped me in the days following Belle's birth. But, truly, she was an amalgamation of all of my nurses who had tended to me so kindly, and with such gentle compassion, during my two hospital stays.

On one hand, I was happy to wake up to my son, the warmth of my bed, the safety of the situation. In that moment, I was not facing an imminent surgery or possibly harrowing delivery. The sky was bright, with sun streaming through my bedroom windows, making colors and shapes appear on the walls.

On the other hand, I felt an extreme sense of loss. In my dream, I had been at the hospital, having our third baby. In my dream, it had been a boy. I'd had a big belly and could feel the shape of my son inside of me—had been able to trace the curves of his spine, like a little railroad track, from the outside. Like everything else in the dream, my ability to feel his body within me had been exaggerated but so tangible. In my dream, there had been such promise.

A few hours later, after our normal Saturday-morning routine of pouring cereal into bowls and juice into glasses and bodies into clothing and love into hugs, my parents called me from some sort of home and design convention. After asking me about couches, and a possible Ping-Pong table, they asked me how I felt about something called "Rent-A-Chicken." A company would come to my house, set up a chicken coop, and provide us with all of the necessary supplies to care for two chickens from April through October, at which time they would come and pick up the chickens for winter. Or something.

"With two chickens," my dad said, "you'll get about fourteen eggs a week, and we would share them with you. We would have fresh eggs, and your yard would be the perfect space for it."

Then he said something I didn't understand—about how the chickens need to be tended to regularly, as after three days they would try to hatch any eggs they had laid. I peppered them with questions, and my anxiety level started to rise. I had wanted to have a chicken coop in my yard for years, and since I have become passionate about gardening and growing vegetables in our greenhouse, I thought that adding fresh eggs to the mix would be wonderful, and healthy, and a great experience for my kids.

"But wait," I started, cautiously. "If we *did not* tend to the eggs after three days, these eggs would hatch? Is that what eggs do? How have I never thought of this before? Are the eggs we eat just little chickens that have yet to develop into chicks? Are the eggs just like ovulation, or are they already fertilized?"

My parents tried to answer, but they really didn't know, either. A hasty Internet search told me that most of the eggs that we buy from the supermarkets are, in fact, unfertilized, yet there are some exceptions, and many of the eggs we buy from farmers' markets are fertilized, and there are ways to tell the difference, either before they are cracked or by certain characteristics shown after.[1]

"I am so confused. What are the yellow chickens we see? I know roosters, because they're the crowing things with the red wattles, but, like, what are hens? In the cartoons, the little hens are brown and have bonnets on, but chickens are yellow, and so I'm lost!"

They laughed, we hung up, and tears started to fill my eyes. Kenny, who had caught the tail end of our conversation, smiled as he asked what crazy scheme my parents and I were concocting and started sending funny text messages and videos to our family's group thread. As I sat, curled up in the white plastic chair in my kitchen, the tears started to soak the knees of my cotton joggers. I was overwhelmed, and what had turned into a happy conversation prompted a cascade of emotions from within me.

"Are you laughing right now, or are you crying?" asked Kenny, still lighthearted in tone as he sent a video message of a rooster head superimposed over his own.

I looked up at him, wordlessly. He saw the tears in my eyes and that they were not tears from belly laughing. He came over to me, sat down on the floor in front of me, and asked me why I was so upset. He questioned me about the chickens and whether I was sad about potentially eating fertilized eggs and reminded me that we almost exclusively eat supermarket eggs, which, as we had learned, are not fertilized.

When I finally looked up at him, with swollen, red eyes and uncontrollable tears, all I could muster was "Can you think of why this might be hard for me?"

In an instant, he got it. He put his hands on my tear-soaked legs and said, "I'm here for you, Bec. I understand."

But despite his incredibly kind sentiment, he could not understand how feverishly my mind was racing—that the conversation about chickens, like so many conversations in my life, morphed from "Fun endeavor!" to "Baby? Baby? Eggs? Baby? Pregnancy? Baby? All the babies?"

I thought about the chickens and how every time they lay an egg that goes unfertilized it is just like every month when I grow a large follicle, housing a fertile egg that is inevitably unused. *My* eggs, that is—not the chickens'. I thought of my reserve of eggs and of all the squandered possibilities. I thought of life being created and how I never wanted to eat a slice of avocado toast topped with a runny egg ever again.

I thought about my dream.

In this mind of mine, all roads lead to baby. Roads that take me to school drop-off. Roads that start out with a visit to the oncology ward. Roads to Rent-A-Chicken.

I thought back to the moment in my dream when Linda and I were in the bathroom and she was lining the toilet seat for me, over and over, and I kept dropping the squares of bath tissue, fumbling around, and delaying the inevitable. My dream was brimming with questions, but my dream also had promise. Possibility. Hope.

I do not yet know whether I will be renting chickens this spring or whether I will be using eggs of any kind (freshly laid in my backyard or created by my ovaries).

It is exhausting.

I want to go back to my dream.

I just want to rest my head and go back to sleep.

Maybe we can.

Three words. Just three simple words that changed everything for me.

In just a few moments, I had gone from suspicious lymph nodes and an uncertain future of bleakness to brimming ovaries and an uncertain future of babyness.

It was as if all of a sudden a bright light were shining down on me, again, as I sat there on the table in my hospital gown and Chanel ballet flats. Possibility colored my cheeks and promise filled my heart.

For me, like it is for many women, the notion of getting pregnant again after suffering from (and surviving) severe perinatal distress is terrifying. It seems, for many, like a set of dominos, each adorned with an "all-or-nothing" demarcation on its face: "Get pregnant again, or no more babies" or "Experience pregnancy again, and experience postpartum depression again" or "I want this badly, and I know I have to walk away." The dominos are perched precariously and with one wrong move they are at risk of falling. And for many of us falling is not an option. We are moms, after all.

But still, there was suddenly a new reality in which I could trade the letters *PPD* for *TTC*—moving from a state of depression to trying to conceive. A reality that we could manifest in which my digital-citizenship profile would morph from images of sad women holding mugs adorned in slogans like "I see you, Mama!" and "#selfcare" to pictures of happy babies and women holding positive pregnancy tests and balloons filled with blue or pink confetti.

In the weeks following my unexpected scare, ultrasound, and hospital visit, my perspective shifted so much that life around me actually looked different. The bright light that I had seen in the hospital continued to shine. Kenny and I talked excitedly about a new baby. I had gone from "No. Zero percent chance" to "Maybe we can" to "I want to try" in what felt like an instant. I believe it was the timing of things. With his mom so ill, Kenny was examining the fragility of life and taking on new perspectives and looking for ways to add joy. And in my heart of hearts, I think he was trying to find a happy distraction.

It was all so abrupt.

It was as if we had taken that magical, yet peaceful, snow globe of my children's lives and shaken it up and the glittery, white pieces had not yet settled back into place. My vision of the life I knew had been obscured by sparkly, shimmering, falling pieces of snow.

Everything changed so suddenly that I could not catch my breath. And when I could, I realized that I had been holding it. I waited for Kenny to change his mind. I asked him, incessantly, if he was sure. Now that he had given this back to me—"this" being the promise of another child—I was petrified of losing it again.

That's when we started with the six purple hearts.

I cannot pinpoint the exact origin of the six purple hearts, but I know that, to me, they meant everything. Kenny and I have always traded texts throughout the day. We talk logistics, and other Married-People Things, but we also send cute messages and lovey messages. And so, during this time, Kenny changed things up. Instead of the typical "kiss-face" emoji or red heart, he started to send me six purple hearts. Purple is my lucky color—so much so that I have to wear purple underwear when I am, or someone I love is, flying. So much so that I made Kenny wear my neon-purple socks into the delivery room for my C-section with Beau, because they would not let me wear them myself. Purple means something.

The six hearts meant even more.

At the time, our family had five members: the two of us, our two children, and our beloved first (fur-st?) child, our Yorkie, Lola.

So when Kenny sent the six hearts to me, he was saying so much more. Kenny. Becca. Belle. Beau. Lola. Baby.

That last heart, that sixth heart, conveyed more than any plain words could. He began to text me six hearts as shorthand for "I love you" or "You mean the world to me" or "We are in this together, forever" or, most important of all, "I am not going to change my mind!"

Six purple hearts, all day, every day.

But of course it wasn't all sunshine emojis and smiley-face emoticons.

The idea of getting pregnant again after my experience with severe prenatal and postpartum depression was so different from my previous pregnancies. Rather than a joyful, eager "mother-to-be-to-be," I felt more like a hybrid of a scientist and investigative journalist, with a dash of med student and sprinkling of interrogator.

The journey and exploration of a future pregnancy post-postpartum made my previous experiences with due-date calculators and those little, cardboard "When was the start of your last menstrual period?" wheels in the OBGYN's waiting room look like—quite literally—child's play. I had to become an expert in fields including (but not limited to) psychology, obstetrics and gynecology, maternal mental health, prescription drugs, surgery, embryology, urology, reproductive endocrinology, and high-risk obstetrics—and in giving myself shots. Many, many, many shots.

But more than the technical parts—and the science parts and even the mental-health parts—this experience felt markedly different to me for one major reason: with my past pregnancies, my parents, family members, and loved ones had been overjoyed. They had been happy to hear when we were "trying" to get pregnant and even more excited when we shared the positive news. As much pain as the notion that I would never be able to have another baby had caused me over the years following Beau's birth, the fellow members of my village had been feeling their own breed of pain. They ached at the thought of me suffering, again. They were still tender in the places they'd been walloped by my illness. Their hearts were still mending.

Once I knew that having another baby was an option, I knew as deeply as one can know that I wanted to try. I just had no idea as to how. I sought answers from any professional I deemed worthy. I needed the physical answers, I needed the psychological answers, and with these I hoped that I would get the thing I needed most: support from the people I loved.

I contacted the hospital where Beau had been born and asked for a copy of my operative reports. After his birth, during my stay in the hospital, I heard the words *adhesions* and *scar tissue* thrown around but had never really explored what they meant for me. I read my report and did follow-up Internet searches for things like "How much blood is considered normal to lose in a cesarean section?" and "What are the risks associated with bladder adhesions?"

And I became informed. I would be my own advocate.

I called the doctors in the hospital's high-risk perinatal group and told them about my situation.

"We no longer deliver babies," one of the nurses told me. "But we do follow women throughout their pregnancies in high-risk situations. And your situation does not seem to be high risk. I don't think the doctors here would even take you on as a patient. You should call your regular OB."

Hearing this news was both comforting and concerning.

In order to find out what would actually be possible for us—me with the adhesions and scar tissue, Kenny with a vasectomy—we made an appointment with a popular fertility specialist practicing in our area. Dr. G, as we call him, is a physician whose expertise has helped couples with fertility issues (in Philadelphia and beyond) bring a lot of babies into this world. We sat in his private office, adorned from floor to ceiling with framed magazine covers and articles extolling his expertise over the years, and my eyes locked on an article about a grandmother who had carried her own grandchild in her uterus.

I made a mental note to text my mom and was just starting to craft the message in my mind when Dr. G walked through his office door, wearing a pair of navy scrubs and a kind, broad smile.

(As an aside, I silently filed away my brilliant "Hey, Mom! How are you? So, just wondering: Would you let someone implant one of my embryos into your uterus so that you could carry a baby for me?" text, noting that it likely needed more finessing than I could spare at the moment.)

Dr. G sat with Kenny and me, listened to our story, gave us the time to voice our concerns, glanced at my operative report, and looked me squarely in the eyes.

"I can talk to you about a million different options right now, but I think you want to have another baby, and you want to carry it. So that's what we're going to do."

Dr. G's tone was warm and his words emphatic.

"You mean I can actually get pregnant again? It is safe for me to carry a baby again?"

He explained to me that while there would be some tall hurdles to jump, he had the right kicks. Not only did he lay out a medical plan for us, but he also put two major caveats in place: First, before he would allow me to get pregnant, I would have to gain enough weight to be considered medically healthy. Second, he would need for all of the members of my psychological treatment team to sign off on the plan, deeming me psychologically stable enough to go through with (or at least try for) another pregnancy. This, to me, was incredibly compassionate health care.

The next meeting was, for me, emotionally challenging in an entirely different way. I had scheduled a sit-down with my OBGYN—the man who had delivered my son, giving me my healthy baby boy. The man who had actually seen what my insides looked like and could give the best analysis of the physical side of things. And the man who had missed diagnosing my postpartum depression and who had sent me home from the hospital with a cheerful suggestion to not have any more children.

What happened wasn't his fault. It wasn't my fault; I didn't *know* to know.

For a long time leading up to this next visit, this hospital had been a very scary place for me. Though I see several specialists there, it is, in many ways, haunted. For years, I would drive onto the property and wince. I would park my car, and I would walk through the dim parking lot into the stairwell, and I would pass pregnant woman after pregnant woman; I would hold their doors and smile at them with an ache in my gut as big as the bulges under their blouses. I would enter through the automatic glass doors of the hospital and pass the outpatient lab on my left, and I would think about the day in 2013 when my ultrasound tech "saw something between the legs" of my fetus during my twelve-week sequential screening scan and how that is when I called my dad to tell him that we were going to be "having a boy!" There were ghosts everywhere.

But this visit would be different. I was not the sad, barren woman whose control had been taken away; rather, I was the optimistic, educated woman whose control had been restored. I would be at the helm of my own ship this time. I could be the one to ask the questions and to lead the

conversation and to gather the data that I needed. I took the elevator to
the third floor of one of the hospital's many buildings and walked down
the hallway that I had not seen for almost four years. The last time I had
been under those rows of fluorescent lighting and popcorn-ceiling tiles, it
was while being pushed in a wheelchair by my mother, on my way to a
postoperative appointment. On that day in 2013 I had looked sallow from
my low hemoglobin levels and burgeoning mental illness. On that day,
my OBGYN had removed the staples from the fresh, angry-looking scar
across my abdomen, and, though it had been too painful and too tiring to
walk normally, my physical feelings had been no match for the turmoil
brewing inside my tormented mind.

And so this new meeting with my OBGYN would end up being as
healing as it was informative. After I arrived at his hospital offices, I was
greeted by his nurse, whom I'd first met in 2009 during my pregnancy
with Belle, and she hugged me like an old friend. I hung out in the back
with her, outside of the exam-room doors, like I was special in some way.
When my doctor returned from a delivery, we sat in his office rather than
in an exam room. Unlike on our other visits, this time we were speaking
on the same level; I was not below him on an exam table, vulnerable in
a gown with my legs in stirrups or my belly exposed. Rather, my doctor
expressed his sympathy for what I had endured and treated me with dignity
in answering my long list of questions.

"Is it safe for me to have another C-section?"

"Well, there would be things about another pregnancy that would make
it a bit more risky, like the scar tissue and your thyroid and with your low
platelets at the end of your pregnancies before, but I'm more worried about
your psychological state and your ability to cope. You have two children
who need you at home."

"Yes, yes," I told him. "I know that, and I have the psychological part
covered. I need to know whether I'm going to die on the table."

He looked at me seriously, without his signature grin and cool attitude.

"If I thought you were going to die on the table, I would tell you not to
do this. I would have to schedule a C-section for you no later than thirty-
eight weeks. I might have to make a completely new incision, internally
and externally. I would have to monitor you closely. But there are some
people whom I advise to not get pregnant again. Physically, if I were worried, I would not let you do this. I won't let anything happen to you."

"And if I get nervous?" I asked.

"You can come in every week for an ultrasound if you need to."

That was all I needed to hear. He was attentive to my emotional needs, he was clear about the physical obstacles, and he was reassuring about my profound fears.

It was only then, after these meetings, and gathering and hoarding data like a little, determined, fertile squirrel, that I presented my proposal to the members of my treatment team. At the time, I had just started with a fantastic new psychologist, I had a standing Tuesday date with my dietitian, and I had semiregular meetings with my psychiatrist, who also doubles as our couple's therapist. To my shock and amazement, no one balked. Don't get me wrong—no one threw a parade with pink and blue balloons adorned to a baby-bottle-shaped-float, but each team member listened to me, expressed their unique concerns, and told me that as long as I was healthy, they would support my decision to expand my family by way of another pregnancy.

There was one universal rule, however, on which we all agreed: the narrative would *not* be "If I have another baby, I will get healthy again!" Rather, it was "If I get healthy again, then I can *try* to have another baby." The distinction would be nuanced in diction and everything in practice.

Our plan would be complex, and it would be fluid. First, we would have to tackle the period of time before I would be deemed ready for pregnancy. Next, my team would work closely with me so that I could have a healthy pregnancy, both physically and emotionally. Finally, my team would be fortified and well prepared for the postpartum period, during which time we would employ all of the coping mechanisms we had been working to master and any new treatment approaches, or medications, if the need did arise.

Our plan was discussed in detail—both in my individual meetings with my team members and in their own phone calls to one another—but it was at a very high level. Instead of going into battle unarmed, like I had before getting pregnant with Beau, I would go into a future pregnancy with skills and support systems and, perhaps most important, reasonable expectations.

For the first part of my "pregnancy plan" (no one called it a *pregnancy plan*, but that's what it was, so that is what it shall be called, henceforth), each team member would have a different role and different requirements, all aimed at leading me to the same goal: physical and mental health. In my weekly therapy sessions with my psychologist—which we had decided to make into longer sessions so that we could get more of the hard work done—we worked to unpack layers of trauma, exorcise the ghosts of my past, and, through trial and error, figure out the tools and strategies that would work best for me. I had worked with a handful of different therapists since my diagnosis with postpartum depression (including psychologists, psychiatrists, and a licensed professional counselor—or LPC—along with family and couple's therapists), but in the spring of 2017 I found my fit. From the start, my psychologist, Dr. S, approached my treatment in a new-to-me way, homing in from previously uncharted angles. She has taught me about boundaries and about how it feels to carry my emotions somatically. She became my coach and has held me accountable. Dr. S is incredibly bright and intuitive, with a razor-sharp memory, and I trust that she knows so much more than I do, which may seem obvious, but I have learned that, though it is absolutely salient for me, it is not a given. Most of all, I trust Dr. S as a person. I like her so very much, and I appreciate her compassion so very much. She has been a gift. She has meant the world to me.

And so, since that time, I have been able to focus on and make so much progress in many different areas of wellness contemporaneously. My team has rallied around me as I work to make my mind resilient and my body strong. But one part of my wellness continues to impede me.

A crucial part of my recovery is centered on my weight, and my weight is a topic I find particularly hard to address. Even mentioning it can be triggering to others, and it is always a sensitive topic, so I feel a tremendous sense of responsibility when broaching the subject. Though I am so open about most aspects of my life, I often dance around the topic of my weight. It scares me. In writing about my physical health, as opposed to my mental health, I have trouble finding the words. It is almost hard to admit this fact:

Since having first been diagnosed with postpartum depression after Beau's birth in October 2013, one of my primary and most identifiable side effects has been my low body weight. My body mass index (BMI) has not been within the normal, healthy range.[2] I have had a problem taking in the proper nutrients and energy that my body needs, attributing this to both physical and mental barriers that seem to have blocked my way. In order to be considered healthy enough to carry a pregnancy, I would need to be at a clinically healthy weight, and yet I've struggled with getting there. It breaks my heart to admit that I have known and lived with this problem with my weight for as long as I have known and lived with my son.

In order to help me with this challenge and others, I have also found an incredible psychiatrist, who is a pillar of my treatment team. Dr. B is brilliant and bold. She is incredibly compassionate and yet appropriately tough on me. She has worked with Kenny and me as a couple, and she has worked with me individually. Her office is filled with curated crafts and art pieces, collected from her trips around the world, and she wears funky jewelry and makes great jokes. She is a force. I adore her, and, more than that, I appreciate her.

Dr. B is also the person responsible for controlling my medication, which is a crucial part of maintaining my mental health. When I first began seeing her in 2015, I was on a pretty strong cocktail of medicines—taking daily an SSRI (Prozac), an aminoketone (Wellbutrin XL), and five milligrams of Klonopin. This last one, Klonopin, is the most noteworthy, because it is a strong benzodiazepine (as well as an antiepileptic drug used, in other cases, to control seizures) and it is contraindicated in pregnancy.

In 2015, the Food and Drug Administration (FDA) changed the way it classifies drug safety in regard to pregnancy, moving from the letter-coding system with which I had become familiar (A, B, C, D, X) to the Pregnancy and Lactation Labeling Final Rule (PLLR), which went into effect on June 30 of that year.[3] Though the new system more comprehensively explicates the medications' effects on pregnancy, it's hard for me to forget the letters to which I had become so accustomed during my two prior pregnancies, before the classification method was modified.

I know that the FDA had labeled Klonopin as a category-D medication, which meant "there *is* positive evidence of human fetal risk based on adverse reaction data from investigational or marketing experience or studies in humans." "But," it had added, "potential benefits may warrant use of the drug in *pregnant* women despite potential risks."[4] Klonopin is not something that I believe I would feel comfortable taking while pregnant. And so as I contemplate a future healthy pregnancy, I know that I have to wean off of the medicine, which I began taking to control my anxiety. This relates directly to second reason why my Klonopin intake is so significant. According to the FDA, while the initial dose for an adult with panic disorder is 0.25 milligrams bid (*bid* stands for the Latin *bis in die*, meaning *two times per day*), "it is possible that some individual patients may benefit from doses of up to a maximum dose of 4 mg/day, and in those instances, the dose may be increased in increments of 0.125 to 0.25 mg bid every 3 days until panic disorder is controlled."[5] Additionally, Klonopin is considered extremely addictive, and the withdrawal, even with the recommended, gradual weaning, can be brutal. To put these numbers into perspective, when I started seeing my psychiatrist, I was taking twenty times the recommended initial dose of this strong medication and more than the highest recommended dose. Since this time I have been slowly weaning off of the Klonopin, and I now take 0.5 milligrams two times a day.

The tricky part in changing my medications is with the antidepressants. To put it in perspective, I had been reluctant to take as much as a single Tylenol capsule during my pregnancy with Belle. With Beau, my arm had to be twisted into taking Zofran, a prescription medication to limit my vomiting to ten times a day. As it stands now, my psychiatrist, psychologist, fertility specialist, obstetrician, husband, and I have all agreed that, for me, staying on my antidepressant medication during a future pregnancy is the wise decision. It is not an easy decision, nor is it a decision with which I am completely at peace. But I know that it is right.

As explained by the Mayo Clinic, studies show that most SSRIs, including Prozac, are considered safe options during pregnancy.[6] Additionally, my bupropion (Wellbutrin) is considered safe, although not typically the first drug prescribed to pregnant women.

Though I have continued to feel confident that should I encounter any prenatal distress in a future pregnancy I would not neglect my fetus or in any way disregard doctors' recommendations, forgoing proper prenatal care, I know that I need to do everything in my power to stay as not-depressed as possible during this time. It is what my husband, children, and family members deserve. It is certainly what any future, growing baby deserves. And though it is hard to write without feeling selfish, it is what I deserve.

A future pregnancy would be unpredictable. All pregnancies are. My plan would morph and change and evolve and grow, in synchronicity with my body. Just like anything in nature, all we can do is to stock up on the proper gear, find the safest place to be, and hold on as tightly as possible. My two pregnancies were so different in so many ways, and so there is no way to write a manual for handling a third. Or, if it were possible, I would make sure to write it in pencil—not in permanent marker or the indelible ink from a printer. I would prescribe continuing my weekly therapy sessions, and if ever I were to stumble, I would have a full mosh pit of people on which to land. I have a feeling that on my mosh pit I could crowd surf to the exact place I'd need to be. I trust my people to hold me up, but I would rather have them hold me up by choice than by necessity. I would like to avoid chaos and cacophony; I would rather have the noise sound like music.

In deciding to explore my options for expanding our family, I was able to take a few more baby steps, while continuing to have countless more baby steps to go.

I read and researched about other women who had taken medicine for their perinatal mood disorders during pregnancy and the postpartum period. I learned in one article for *The Atlantic* that "since many antidepressants, in limited testing, show a low risk to fetuses, doctors often let pregnant people choose what they want to do. There isn't a wealth of information on the subject because almost no one wants to test drugs on pregnant or nursing parents. You cannot Google your way to the right answer. This means that these decisions cannot be made based just on facts. They have to be made largely on priorities. The thing is, there is no way to be risk-averse while pregnant. Being pregnant is itself a life condition that is inherently risky." The article's author, Liz Tracy, also shared the stories of other women, many of whom work in health care, who, when faced with this dilemma, decided to stay on antidepressants during their pregnancies, as it was deemed the better choice.[7]

I was arming myself with every bit of knowledge I could, but I knew my arduous trek was only just beginning. When it came to my family members and closest friends, I would have a steeper, more bramble-covered mountain to climb. Those closest to me—along with those not close to me—knew how much I had been struggling with my inability to expand my family. It was something that was with me all the time, and I had been doing a poor job of hiding it, when I even tried.

But I was doing due diligence. I would come to my loved ones from a position of strength. And yet it was still terrifying. Each and every time.

First I spoke to my parents. They were, understandably, standoffish. The subject, for them, was like being close to a glowing fire: It can be mesmerizing and feels so warm, and the closer you get, the warmer and warmer and warmer it feels and the brighter and brighter and brighter it looks. But the line between allure and peril is so very thin. Before you know it, you are burning, licked with flames, and simply trying to survive.

I think my mom and dad had to compartmentalize the news. Kenny and I told them that we had visited a fertility doctor and would be using science to create embryos as an insurance policy of sorts—that, with age on my side, we would simply go through the first part of in vitro fertilization (IVF), make embryos, freeze them, and, maybe, use them at a later date if and when I was deemed healthy and if and when it was the right decision for our family. As parents, they want for me to be happy and they want for me to be healthy, and those things are not always congruent. They were supportive of our idea—but from a distance. The burns they had suffered during my severe postpartum depression had finally healed, and they had only just gotten their lives back. They would watch the fire but from a balcony above us. It would be different this time because it had to be.

My sister, Emily, had the same mixed feelings. She displays her vulnerability more quietly than I do. When we were growing up, I took up so much airspace in our lives that it was often hard for her to sneak in a word. It was not that she felt less; she just felt what she felt more quietly—differently. Today, as an incredibly successful journalist and author, Emily has a strong voice that she uses to help many and to guide our country. I knew I might not get her approval with my news, but I wanted her to not actively disapprove of the idea. She peppered me with a number of questions, like the seasoned reporter she is, and pointed out all of the possible pitfalls. She also questioned me about why I felt another child was necessary. This, I know, was out of pure love and concern for me, Kenny, my parents, and my kids. In the end I got her to buy into the we-are-making-embryos-just-to-have-in-case-we-want-to-use-them-down-the-line logic, and that was good enough for me.

My friends are crucial parts of my support system, the ones who stepped in and helped me with my children when I could not do it myself. They have held me and coached me and given me bountiful compassion and tough love and all the things you hope your best friends will give you. As I always say, my tribe is the best tribe.

I talked to Kim and Jess in person, and I think they were both shocked. They are my oldest and dearest friends, and we talk every single day—in person, on the phone, or, most often, in our ongoing group text thread, titled "The Chat Room"—about subjects ranging from baby poop to recipes for soup to medical worries to outfit choices to current events to past memories and so much more. We have known each other forever—Kim and I since we were six years old and in the same first-grade class, and Jess and I since we were sixteen years old and with the same eleventh-grade English teacher. We danced at each other's weddings and have leaned on each other through our woes. We have held each other's babies, and Kim and Jess have definitely held my hair back during some particularly "festive" nights out. We have seen each other through so many things. We have established a code, whereby "100 percent best-friend honesty" can be applied to a question or as a statement. If you ask for 100 percent best-friend honesty, it means you have posed a very tough question, knowing the answer could be painful, but brutal truth is required. If invoking 100 percent best-friend honesty, it means you are being as truthful as one can be. They knew my pain, and so I did not need to explain why having another baby is so important to me.

Their reactions to my news were clear and kind and the same: They both said that they wanted me to be happy and that they knew how much I had been longing for another baby. But they were adamant that I be as healthy as possible, both physically and mentally, before I became pregnant or in any way expanded my family. They want me to be content in my life, but, even more than that, they want me to be *alive* in my life.

I approached only a few other best friends with this tough topic, receiving the same support from each one. When I told Erin, my other half—whom I have written about as "Twin" for years on my blog, as we share a birthday (and oh so much more!)—she smiled her enormous smile and nodded her approval; as long as I was healthy and the doctors were on board, she would be thrilled for me. I told Brooke, my soul friend, over text, and she wrote effusively, with exclamation points and happy faces; like everyone else I told, Brooke took this news very seriously, as she has been privy to the depths of my pain, and she said she supported me 100 percent and just wanted for me to be well. Each time I told a close friend about this "maybe-baby" idea, I felt scared, whether it was cuddled up on a familiar couch during a weekly chai date or curled up in the booth of a restaurant over spicy margaritas. And though I fielded different, nuanced questions from my friends, the same sentiment was echoed over and over again—support and wishes for my health and joy.

The last two people whom I felt, at the time, we needed to consult were perhaps the most important individuals of all: Belle and Beau. Aside from Kenny, our decision would change no one's life more than theirs, and I needed to know where they stood on the issue of another sibling.

Belle had so eloquently comforted me in my not-so-well-hidden grief, years prior, by telling me that I was a tree.

This had happened on one afternoon when I was driving my kids home from a long day of school, back when she was five and Beau was one. The subject of babies had been broached. Belle could see the emotion swelling in me, even from her perch in her car seat in the back of my car.

"You already have your fruit, Mom," she said. "You are a tree. You made two pieces of fruit. You made my brother and me. And that is the fruit that your tree is supposed to make."

How would she feel about another apple being added, first to me, then into our barrel?

I needed to know. I convinced myself that I needed to know for their sakes, but, in hindsight, I think it was more for my own.

And this is where we made a big mistake. A #parentingfail, so to speak. In our eagerness to share our anticipation and elation with the kids, Kenny and I unthinkingly exposed them to a lot of potential disappointment. Nothing was a given. But in the moment, our only focus was on the joy and eagerness we hadn't let ourselves entertain for too many years. We simply got caught up in all of the excitement.

I don't remember exactly how we broached the subject of another baby, but once we got an enthusiastic "Yes! Yes, please! Please, have another baby, please, please!" response from both kids, we began to feel, and show, the same level of zeal.

At the time, it felt, to them, that having another baby was our choice and so if we decided to do it, it would be done—they'd have another little apple, and it would only serve to sweeten our bunch.

I got swept away by this enthusiasm, and we began talking, openly and often, about a new baby. Both Belle and Beau expressed their desire for me to have a baby boy. Beau wanted the chance to have a brother; Belle loved having a little brother already and, as she admitted, did not want another girl in the family who could possibly steal any of her feminine thunder. The four of us talked, giddily, about how we would announce a pregnancy to the world.

"Maybe we should be superheroes," Beau suggested.

"Actually, I kind of like that idea!" I enthused. "We could all dress up and say something like 'They told us it was impossible, but . . .' and then hold up a sign."

The kids dreamed up ideas for a "gender-reveal" party, like they had heard about from friends or seen in Instagram videos. We agreed that, despite our belief in our house that every color is for every person, in this case pink would stand for a girl and blue for a boy, just to make it easier for everyone. They vacillated between cupcakes with colored centers, a huge box filled with balloons that would fly out, and more outlandish ideas, involving things like paintball guns and exploding baseballs.

The details didn't matter to me. All that mattered was that this baby was already being embraced by our little family, and I felt so much less self-ish about the endeavor, seeing how excited my children were for a new sibling. Belle assured me that she would get up in the middle of the night for the baby's feedings. I assured Beau that a baby would not chew up and ruin his Star Wars toys. We were intoxicated with joy. With hope.

I kept a running list of baby names in a note on my phone and would add and change names every hour. I would look up names and their meanings.

I would write out our names, along with new possible name options to see how they all flowed together.

Love, Becca, Kenny, Belle, Beau, and

Love, Rebecca, Kenny, Annabelle, Alexander Beau, and

Annabelle, Alexander, and

Belle, Beau, and

With love and joy, parents Rebecca and Kenny, along with big sister Belle and big brother Beau, welcome

It was never-ending.

My baby steps had turned into daring leaps.

With our medical and personal-support teams on board, we were able to really start down our Dreft-scented path. We had come to the conclusion that our first choice when it came to family expansion was for me to try to create and carry a baby biologically, through IVF. It had been deemed safe by a team of experts and in many ways felt natural despite its being completely unnatural in many others. In terms of how to bring a baby into the world, pregnancy is all I've ever (personally) known.

The fertility specialist gave us a plan of action, having considered all of the physical, emotional, and financial factors we set forth. Because of my age and fertility (both the blood test used to measure my hormone levels, along with egg quality, and the internal ultrasounds done to look at my ovaries confirmed a strong-looking egg reserve), we would qualify for different studies being run by drug companies. This would help us defray some of the expenses associated with IVF and also afford us more information than we would have otherwise.

I qualified for a study designed to determine the efficacy of one ovary-stimulating drug versus another, in which I would be given a randomly assigned drug used to stimulate my ovaries so that instead of producing one egg during a cycle, they would produce many. Instead of reversing Kenny's vasectomy (a procedure that is not always effective, is extremely costly, takes a significant amount of time before its success can be evaluated, and, not for nothing, would leave him *without* a vasectomy), a urologist would harvest sperm directly from his testicles. This (very unpleasant procedure) would involve a needle aspiration from his epididymis or, if no sperm could be collected by this less invasive method, a testicular biopsy, where tissue would be removed from the inside of his testicle, the sperm then harvested directly from there.

As dictated by the study, I would be placed on an oral birth-control pill for a month leading up to my stimulating cycle and then would be

monitored at the fertility clinic, with blood work and a transvaginal ultrasound, every other day. During this time, I would be injecting myself
at home with the stimulating medicine, and the nurses would watch my
hormone levels rise and follicle numbers grow until the doctor deemed it
an appropriate time to trigger ovulation.

Then I would give myself an injection of HCG (human chorionic go-
nadotropin, more commonly known as "the pregnancy hormone") and then
another medication to stop my body from ovulating on its own. Exactly
thirty-six hours after my HCG injection, both Kenny and I would arrive
at the fertility clinic, where his sperm and my eggs would be retrieved.
Embryologists would analyze both my eggs and his sperm and collect the
best of each on which to perform intracytoplasmic sperm injection (ICSI),
the manual injection of an individual sperm into an individual egg.

With ICSI, my doctor explained to us, fertilization rates typically range
from 50 to 80 percent, and then any fertilized eggs would be kept in a safe,
temperature-controlled, light-controlled space. Any potential embryos created would be monitored for five days (with progress reports given to us
on days three and five) to see whether they were dividing properly, how
they looked to the trained eye of the embryologist, and what their "grades"
would be (a measure of their quality).

On day five, as part of the study, all viable embryos would be biopsied
for preimplantation genetic screening (PGS), a process by which the embryos would have a few cells microsurgically removed and then screened
for chromosomal abnormalities. The embryos would then be frozen and
stored while we would wait for the results.

That was how it was *supposed* to go.

In reality, as is often the case, it did not go exactly as planned or, unfor-
tunately for us, as hoped.

What actually happened? A shit show.

On May 31, 2017, our ninth wedding anniversary, my phone rang at four
in the afternoon. It was my husband, on his way home from work early, as
we had planned to go out for a special anniversary dinner.

"The nursing home just called," his voice broke. "My mom has taken
a turn."

He went on to explain to me that not only was my mother-in-law no
longer lucid, but she was also no longer conscious. The nurse had told him
that while she expected his mother to live through the weekend, she would
not live to see the next. My heart fell to my feet. I thought of our visit to
Susan's condo on Valentine's Day, just a few months prior, and how she

and I had debated the merits of gray paint. (She did not care for it, and I reminded her that, aside from white, it was the color that I had used for every room in my house.)

How could she be dying?

Kenny rallied. "I still want to go out to dinner," he said.

"Love," I was quiet, yet steadfast with my tone. "We are not going to dinner tonight. We are going to be with your mom."

We spent the night of our ninth anniversary in Susan's room at her nursing home, with Kenny on the chair next to her and me cuddled up on the bed, right at her feet. She was not conscious and had not had anything to eat or drink in days, but I talked to her nonetheless.

"Of course you had to make this day about you!" I joked to her, the small, fragile shell of the elegant, beautiful woman I once knew. I rambled on about the fertility doctor and future plans. About how we wanted to have another baby and knew she would have concerns but that she shouldn't worry.

I had known Susan since I was twenty years old, and although I could not honestly say that she was a second mother to me, she had become a very important person in my life. I was—and would always be—the closest thing that she would ever have to a daughter, and that meant something to both of us.

Kenny and I stayed with her until nearly eleven o'clock that night and then went home, where we ate frozen burritos in front of the television in our living room.

Kenny apologized for having to miss out on our anniversary dinner.

"What do you think marriage is all about?" I asked him, rhetorically. "It's about *this*. Sickness and health. Being there for each other. This is real love."

The next week felt like it trudged on for months. I wish that I could say it was a blur in my mind, but I still remember it so vividly and with so much pain. I spent every day with Susan, holding her hand, singing to her, telling her stories, fixing her hair, coating her lips with Vaseline and, when I knew there would be visitors, her coral lipstick. She remained unconscious and was kept comfortable, thanks to the members of the hospice team, for whom I had become the primary point of contact. On one of the days that I was left alone with her in the room, I took her hand in my own and leaned in, placing my face next to hers.

"You know we are going to have another baby." I shared more of our secret with her, as we had decided to start the first part of the IVF process that month. "We'll name the baby for you."

I promised her this and that I would take care of her son. I asked her to be our angel, to watch over and protect us and our children and this baby that had not yet been made. And then I encouraged her to let go.

True to form, she stayed stubborn until the end, and true to the nurse's prediction, she made it through the first weekend but not to the next. On her last day alive, she and I sat together, alone, for the entire morning. I sang to her.

I sang her favorite music, like the Rolling Stones and Bob Seger and the Beatles' song "In My Life," which was the song that she and Kenny had danced to at our wedding. Finally, I sang "Somewhere Over the Rainbow" and kissed the translucent skin on her forehead one last time. At five o'clock the next morning, we got the call that we had been both anticipating and dreading: Susan had passed away and was finally at peace.

That very same day, I got my period. This meant that my IVF cycle was officially starting, and the symbolism was not lost on me. I took it as a good sign.

Per the study protocol, I started on a very low dose of oral birth-control pills and began the monitoring process. As one life ended, I thought, another life would be beginning. Her spirit would be going into our future child. Though I knew that I would not be implanting our embryo immediately, it was exciting to think that we would be making and freezing and storing embryos, especially while I had my age on my side. I was thirty-two years old.

In July 2017, I began my stimulating cycle and was randomly assigned to take a drug called Menopur. Every evening I would formulate my medicine with a mixture of saline and powder, sterilize my stomach, and inject myself with the ovary stimulator. Every other day I would visit the office for blood tests and internal ultrasounds, and at each appointment the nurse would have me write down numbers for each follicle on each ovary. Together we watched as they grew, in number and in size, and everything looked great. After eleven days of stimulating shots, I was finally deemed ready for my HCG injection. This is done with a bigger needle, and, as opposed to being a little shot like the ones I had been giving myself at home, it is an intramuscular injection, straight into the butt cheek. That morning—a Saturday—the nurse even drew a circle, in purple marker, on my butt, to show me where Kenny should do the honors.

This shot, they explained, was too hard for me to do myself. And the timing had to be precise. Because my retrieval was scheduled for 8 A.M. the following Monday, the trigger shot had to be administered at exactly

8 P.M. that Saturday. And because of the way that life works, that Saturday night I had a rock concert to put on. That is not a metaphor. Rather, my long-time music partner and I had been booked as the opening act that evening for an outdoor Dar Williams show.

As we drove to the 5 P.M. sound check for our concert, where I would be singing and dancing around on stage, I explained that I was carrying my kid's lunchbox with me to serve as a thermos for my coconut water, vitamin water, watermelon water, water, and preloaded HCG syringe.

Our show went off without a hitch, and after belting out "Angel from Montgomery" and the rest of our set list, we got back into the car and drove to meet his family, where I scurried to their bathroom. It was there that I contorted my body so that I could administer the HCG injection into my *own* butt cheek, sticking the long, thick needle in as far as it would go. I messed something up the first time, and so I had to try to fill the syringe up again in order to collect all of the liquid and then give myself the painful shot a second time. Alone, in the master bathroom of my friends' house. Life can be so weird sometimes.

The morning of our egg-retrieval procedure, Kenny and I woke up anxious and eager and rode quietly in an Uber to the fertility clinic where I had spent so much of the past month. By this point, my ovaries felt like heavy grapefruits inside of me, and I was eager to find some relief. We were both given anesthesia through ports in our arms, and when we woke up we were in an adjoining room, behind a double set of curtains. The last time I had shared a similar makeshift suite had been during my darkest of days, when Beau had developed respiratory syncytial virus (RSV) at two months old and he and I shared a suite in the emergency room. My mind flashed back to that trying moment, but I did my best to tuck it back neatly into my amygdala and brought myself back to the present-day-embryo-making situation. Like I said, life can be so weird sometimes.

Kenny's urologist came in first. He informed us that the procedure had been harder than anticipated; he could not retrieve enough sperm with the needle aspiration, and so he'd had to do the testicular biopsy. And even with those extra measures, Kenny, like all men who have had a vasectomy, had sperm that had not yet gone through the maturation process and therefore were not the best quality. They would work with what they had and hope for the best.

My doctor was the next to pay us a visit. They had retrieved twenty mature eggs from me and were very optimistic. My ovaries were very large, and so I would be given medicine to "shut down my system" and allow my body to reset. I was showing signs of ovarian hyperstimulation syndrome (OHSS), which, in its worst cases, could be deadly, and so I was given explicit instructions to rest, stay hydrated, and eat as much salty animal protein as I could handle. The irony of it all was that because of my mild OHSS I appeared five months pregnant, a cruel joke of nature. And because we were still keeping this plan very close to our vests, I could not tell anyone why I was waddling around, wearing flowy tops and clutching my pelvis.

The next morning, I got my first of many surprising phone calls from a member of the embryology team. She informed me that they had performed ICSI on fifteen of my twenty eggs and that of those fifteen, five fertilized. Using some quick mental math, I realized that only one-third of the eggs they'd injected had fertilized (and only a quarter of the eggs they had retrieved), which seemed far lower than the 50–80 percent success rate that had been predicted. I was surprised, if not disappointed, but I kept my mind focused on the five little eggs that could.

On day three, while was at the fertility clinic for an OHSS check, I received another call. The embryologist rattled off a bunch of numbers to me, explaining that all five embryos were still looking viable but that some had divided into six cells, some into eight, and one into twelve. Because I had a captive audience of nurses and study coordinators, I asked each of them the same questions:

"Is this a good sign? Do embryos that make it to day three usually continue to thrive? Is the biggest hurdle getting from fertilization to day three?"

Every person assured me that, yes, this was a good sign; that, yes, the eggs should continue to thrive; and that, yes, the numbers seemed great.

One of the kind nurses ushered me into a darkened ultrasound room, and when I instinctively put my legs into the stirrups, she told me that I could sit back—this would be an external ultrasound.

She wanted to make sure my ovaries were shrinking appropriately and that no excess follicular fluid was leaking elsewhere in my body. Normally this kind of ultrasound would have given me pangs, just as it had months earlier in the cancer unit at the hospital. But this time it felt different, and this time I thanked my previously forsaken fertility as the nurse was able to assure me that everything was looking good. I envisioned a future in which I would, once again, have the wand gliding across the warm gel on my belly, squinting to spot tiny, precious baby body parts.

It was on day five that things started to take a real turn. When the embryologist called, she informed me that only two of the embryos had made it; the others had arrested or appeared completely abnormal. The two remaining embryos would be the ones biopsied for the PGS, and I would be notified with the results in approximately two weeks.

Twenty eggs retrieved, fifteen hand-injected with Kenny's sperm, five fertilized, two remaining. The numbers were extraordinary, but not in the way I'd hoped. Every day was agonizing as I waited for my test results, and as I stared into the faces of my beautiful children, I couldn't help but picture them with a new little sibling. I thought of newer, even more creative ways in which we could announce a future pregnancy. I bought a three-pack of onesies too cute to resist.

I don't know what time it was when the embryologist finally called nearly two weeks later, but I do remember it being dark; I'm not sure whether it was dark outside or if that's just how the world began to look to me, but when I picture it now, I see darkness.

I sat alone on the sofa in my living room, and I held my breath, waiting and praying.

She told me, in a tone that did not reflect any emotion, that I had one chromosomally healthy embryo. The other, she explained, had three different chromosomal abnormalities that were "not compatible with life."

I heard the words *monosomy* and *trisomy*, and my brain stopped working.

It was missing chromosomes in places where a chromosome should be and had extras in places where they shouldn't.

"Why does that happen?" I asked, fighting back the deluge of tears that wanted to erupt from a place deep inside of my being. "Everyone said these embryos looked so perfect."

"Sometimes these things just happen," she explained without really giving me an explanation or solace or understanding.

And then there was one.

With only one successfully fertilized egg in the bank, eight months later Kenny and I tried another round of IVF, using the same medicine but with me stimulating for only eight days to avoid another OHSS situation. Once again, everything looked great on my end. Great follicles growing steadily, a pillowy uterus thickening daily. To address Kenny's sperm issues, he saw a different urologist, who put him on medicine to help the sperm quality. During the retrieval procedure, this time Kenny's doctor was able to get enough sperm with just a needle aspiration, and he said they looked good. They had so much, in fact, that they were able to freeze a vial. I hugged the doctor when he delivered the good news.

On my end, Dr. G retrieved another ten strong-looking eggs from my ovaries.

"I promise you that we will get you pregnant," he said. He was very happy with how everything looked. "I wouldn't have come in on this gross, rainy morning if I weren't as confident as I am."

The next morning, when the embryologist called, I knew from her voice that it was not good news. Only one egg had fertilized. By day five none of the eggs had matured into blastocysts. I had no embryos to send for testing. It was a failed cycle, entirely.

Two rounds of IVF, thirty retrieved eggs, all of the things done right, and we were left with one embryo. One.

> One little embryo, sitting all alone,
> Frozen in the clinic, until it finds its home.

4

❖ ❖

Blueprints: Pregnancy After Postpartum Depression

As I shared in my first book, in which I chronicled my journey with severe prenatal and postpartum anxiety and depression, postpartum depression affects approximately 9–13 percent of pregnant women. However, since my book's publication in late 2017, the number of reported cases of postpartum depression has grown to approximately 10–20 percent according to multiple sources, including the Illinois Department of Public Health.[1] "Additionally," as I explained in my first book, "pregnant women can suffer from anxiety, panic attacks, obsessions and compulsions, post-traumatic stress disorder, and other psychological disorders."[2]

I say this with the utmost humility, but every time I give a speech or presentation, I walk off the stage and am, inevitably, greeted with indescribable warmth and, more important, stories. Every time.

When I walked from the huge podium in front of the United States Capitol Building on the National Mall during the 2018 March for Moms, where I was one of only two speakers talking about maternal *mental* health, I was met by so many people who hugged me and thanked me and shared with me. After embracing my kids, parents, and Kenny, I was greeted by some of the other speakers of the day, who had left their spots in the comfort of the VIP tent to meet me. A woman who was there to talk about her near-death experience with postpartum preeclampsia hugged me, held both of my forearms in her hands, and looked at me, right into my eyes.[3]

"Thank you," she said. "This happened to me, too." I had similar interactions with several of the other speakers, and then I walked toward the crowd to watch the rest of the presentation.

It was then that a young woman came up to me and enveloped me into a tearful hug.

"My family wants to meet you," she said, tears glistening on her cheeks. "We lost my sister, Emily, to postpartum depression."

She then did me the honor of introducing me to her family that was there with her that day. I met and embraced each one of them, and they told me about Emily, the beloved daughter, the beloved sister, whose life had been taken from them by postpartum depression. I was able to hug and to comfort Emily's parents. Her siblings. And Emily was not. None of this was lost on me.

And this has continued to happen. Early in 2019, when I stepped off the stage at the Women's March on Philadelphia, shivering from the frigid January cold, one of the event coordinators essentially scooped me up into a giant bear hug. When we broke contact, I saw that she had a line of tears from each of her eyes, streaming straight down her face, and it all seemed so surreal.

"My daughter went through this," she said. "I had no idea. I didn't understand. Now I understand." Her emotions were contagious, and I welled up with tears myself. She thanked me, and then she turned to my mom, who was there, along with my dad, Kenny, and kids. They were part of a sisterhood of a different kind, and they hugged in unspoken kinship.

This same thing has happened time and time again, and it is not because of me or my story or how I tell it; it is because postpartum depression impacts so many people, and I am just a personification of the pain that so many know so intimately, so intensely.

This is why the question of pregnancy after postpartum depression is nuanced, and it is heavy.

The topic has been researched, studied, and discussed, but even with its relatability, I have only been able to find one book dedicated to the topic. Karen Kleiman, a true expert and prolific author in the field of perinatal psychological issues, published a book in 2005 titled *What Am I Thinking? Having a Baby after Postpartum Depression.* Kleiman explains, "[Women are] telling me how much they've been through, how strong they feel for the most part and how terrified they feel about having another baby."[4] Her work is comprehensive, and it is helpful, and it is filled with practical, actionable advice for mothers and their family members (even including a husband's perspective). But it was written more than a decade ago, and the data have changed. So while Kleiman's book is a valuable resource and part of any well-stocked library on pregnancy and postpartum depression, and I'm so grateful to have my copy, we need more, and more recent, information to help guide women making this choice.

Among those of us considering pregnancy after postpartum depression, I fall into a particular subcategory: What happens when someone wants to expand her family after postpartum depression and needs to seek out fertility treatments to do so? In other words, the intricacy of issues to consider when a woman wants another child after the hell of severe postpartum depression is only complicated when she is so determined that she is willing to use fertility treatments—those that are extremely expensive and potentially risky—just to achieve another pregnancy. Does this happen often? Statistically speaking, no.

But it happened to me.

The symptoms of postpartum depression are, in fact, almost identical to those of generalized depression. Postpartum depression, however, is the occurrence of diagnosable depressive disorder after the birth of a child. According to the American Psychological Association, for nearly half of the women who are diagnosed with postpartum depression, this is the first time they are diagnosed with depression in their lifetime.[5]

The risk factors for perinatal distress are, in many ways, intuitive and, in many ways, extremely relevant to the decision to expand one's family (or not). As I wrote in *Beyond the Baby Blues*, "the most significant risk factor for prenatal distress is a woman's history of anxiety, depression, or other mental health problems," and this is still true today. "If a woman has experienced perinatal issues in the past (with prenatal distress, postpartum depression, or both), then she has a much higher risk for a recurrence during a subsequent pregnancy."[6]

"Women who have battled postpartum depression in one pregnancy are more at risk for its return in a later pregnancy," writes Madeline R. Vann, MPH. "So, naturally, many moms wonder if having a second child is worth it."[7]

This increased risk for a recurrence of postpartum depression ranges from 30 percent, among those who have previously suffered from one episode of postpartum depression, to 70 percent, among those women who suffered from postpartum psychosis. Women with a history of postpartum bipolar depression have a 50 percent increased risk of recurrence in a subsequent pregnancy.[8]

What does one do when she has weighed the risks, studied the statistics, consulted with her treatment team, searched her soul, and decided to try to carry a pregnancy, again, after having suffered from perinatal distress?

The first line of defense is a high-level, holistic approach to health care. Generally, the ideal scenario for a postpartum depression survivor entering into a subsequent pregnancy is one in which she has a support team in place, composed of family members, professionals, and anyone else who might fortify her on her quest.

On the personal side, we know that so many women feel tremendous guilt about their prenatal or postpartum anxiety and depression, and so having compassionate, gentle ports in the storm, so to speak, can provide tremendous comfort.

A woman who perceives herself as being inadequate is in a great deal of pain. For a woman with children who thinks she's a bad mother, the mental anguish can be unbearable. Every activity can prove challenging, from each diaper change to every feeding. Trying to engage in her own self-care activities, like showering and brushing her teeth, can be equally burdensome. Cheerful affirmations, even when incredibly well intentioned, can be as palatable as bile.

And the debilitating effects of a chronically low self-esteem can be one of the worst things that a pregnant woman can experience.

Clinically, there are multiple approaches to treating mood disorders in women during pregnancy and the postpartum period. Dr. Amy Wenzel specializes in cognitive behavioral therapy but also uses techniques from dialectical behavior therapy, trauma treatment, and psychotherapy to treat her patients. She worked with me as I compiled data for my first book, sharing information and stories with me from clinical cases. I learned that talk therapy may not be a sufficient intervention for some women suffering mood disorders during pregnancy, and they may require medication.

For many women, this can be upsetting, as they do not want to put anything foreign or chemical in their bodies while they are pregnant. In some cases, a woman has to decide whether to stay on her anxiety or depression medication during her pregnancy, or whether she can find other ways to cope without it. In other cases, women without preexisting mental health conditions may be encouraged to start taking medication in an effort to regulate their emotions.

Because of this conflict, one that is both internal and external, psychological and medical, the American Psychiatric Association and the American College of Obstetricians and Gynecologists teamed up to write a comprehensive report on the use of medication—specifically antidepressants—during pregnancy. Their goal was "to address the maternal and neonatal risks of both depression and antidepressant exposure and develop algorithms for periconceptional and antenatal management." . . . "Both depression symptoms and the use of antidepressant medications during pregnancy have been associated with negative consequences for the newborn. Infants born to women with depression have increased risk for irritability, less activity and attentiveness, and fewer facial expressions compared with those born to mothers without depression. Depression and its symptoms are also associated with fetal growth change and shorter gestation periods. And while available research still leaves some questions unanswered, some studies have linked fetal malformations, cardiac defects, pulmonary hypertension, and reduced birth weight to antidepressant use during pregnancy." . . . Approximately 13 percent of pregnant women have reported taking an antidepressant at some point during their pregnancy. . . .

"Ob-gyns are the front-line physicians for most pregnant women and may be the first to make a diagnosis of depression or to observe depressive symptoms getting worse. In the past, reproductive-health practitioners have felt ill-equipped to treat these patients because of the lack of available guidance concerning the management of depressed women during pregnancy. . . . This joint report bridges the gap by summarizing current research on various depression treatment methods and can assist clinicians in decision-making. Many people—physicians and women alike—will be glad to know that their choices go beyond 'medication or nothing.'"[9]

Echoing the insights of the American Psychiatric Association and American College of Obstetricians and Gynecologists, Christine Dunkel Schetter and Lynlee Tanner point to severe risk factors for both mother and child, stemming from anxiety, depression, and stress during pregnancy: "Anxiety in pregnancy is associated with shorter gestation and has adverse implications for fetal neurodevelopment and child outcomes."[10]

In summary, researchers in the fields of both medicine and psychology have found that the less anxious and distressed a woman is during her pregnancy, the better the outcome will be for her and her baby. Keeping in mind risk factors for physical- and mental-health conditions for both the mother and the fetus, it is important that a woman's prenatal distress be managed appropriately. Ideally this can be done through proper diagnosis, support, and therapy. In other, more severe cases, pregnant women can take antidepressant medications prescribed by their physicians when it is indicated that the risk of depression outweighs any possible risk to her growing baby. It is a balancing act, but with continued research, increased awareness, a commitment to compassionate health care, and additional comprehensive studies on maternal, fetal, and pediatric health, women can be set up for and guided through successful prenatal and postpartum periods.[11]

Pregnancy after prenatal and postpartum anxiety and depression can be safe, and it can be unsafe. It can be uneventful, and it can be ugly. We cannot control the outcome of our stories, but we can do our best to arm ourselves with knowledge, tools, support, and the profound sense of autonomy that so many of us lose to our mental illnesses. While no two stories of pregnancy after perinatal distress are alike, the same can be said for a nonclinically significant pregnancy.

As helpful as the research literature is, I sought out answers from real women who had been in the trenches like I had—women who had battled postpartum depression or other mental health disorders and decided to forge ahead, with or without trepidation, to expand their families. They bravely share their stories with me—and us—in their own written words and illustrate that while biologically having a baby beyond the blues is not always easy, it is most certainly possible.

BRIERLEY, THIRTY-SIX YEARS OLD

I still have both of the photos on my iPhone. November 18, 2014. The first one is of a positive pregnancy test resting atop my bathroom vanity. The second is a grinning, slightly teary-eyed selfie. This was my sixth pregnancy, and as with the previous five, I was elated to see those two pink lines.

But also, as with each pregnancy that followed my very first, I was incredibly nervous.

But let me back up a few years, to the end of 2012.

My first two pregnancies had ended early in miscarriages. My third pregnancy brought me my first daughter. She was born with two congenital anomalies, which we did not discover until her one-week visit to the pediatrician, and a few weeks later I was diagnosed with postpartum depression.

The diagnosis came during one of my early follow-up appointments with my OBGYN. I sat in the exam room alone, which was a first since delivery, and through a constant stream of tears, I recounted to her all that I had learned about my daughter's diagnoses. I told her, too, that I was crying a lot at home and that my mother was staying with us because my husband was back at work, which meant traveling overseas. I don't think we discussed much else—like the fact that I had completely lost my appetite and so my mom was forcing me to eat ice cream for dinner, just to get calories into my body, or that I didn't want any of my friends to come over to meet my baby, even though I'm typically extremely social. My doctor did not ask me whether I thought about hurting myself or my baby girl. (I didn't, though.) She recommended I try a low dose of an antidepressant, wrote me a prescription, and went down the hall to see her next patient. This would be my first time on an antidepressant, but I knew I had to try.

A few days later when I was at a follow-up appointment with my daughter's pediatrician, the doctor looked at me with deep sympathy in his eyes and asked, softly, how I was doing. It was an open-ended question, and his face betrayed no look that he expected a particular answer from me. Still, I robotically explained the emotions I'd been experiencing and told him that I had just started taking Zoloft. He then suggested I also try talk therapy and gave me the name of someone who specialized in postpartum depression.

It took a little bit of time for me to get onto the therapist's schedule. And when the day of my appointment eventually arrived, I had only a very short commute: I rode the elevator down just one floor from the children's unit to her offices. The appointment fell the day after my daughter's first surgery. I had zero expectations for that first visit; I still lacked an appetite, I was crying less but still often, I had not rebounded socially at all, and I wanted to sleep whenever I could. In that first session, my therapist validated all of my feelings. She told me my thoughts and fears and emotions were normal. I left feeling supported and hopeful and stronger.

I desperately needed that strength. And from there my husband and I devoted the first year of our daughter's life to "fixing" the combined three diagnoses—my postpartum depression and our daughter's congenital anomalies. We interviewed doctors, learned about her course of treatment, and scheduled the four surgeries she needed in the first six months of life. Meanwhile, I took my daily dose of Zoloft and continued weekly therapy sessions.

At the six-month mark—March 2013—my daughter sailed successfully through her fourth and final surgery. Shortly after that, under my therapist's supervision, I started to wean off the Zoloft. And just as summer came into full swing, my therapist and I parted ways. But not without a much-needed security blanket: her door was always open to me; I could come back at any time, she told me.

My daughter's first birthday was a joyous occasion. We had what felt like so much more to celebrate than other typical first-time parents did by the time we reached that one-year mark. We had done right by her medically, and despite her early obstacles, she was completely on track developmentally for her age by all measures, checking all the right boxes at each of her doctor check-ins.

I "beat" my postpartum depression and had a new, shiny tool kit to use whenever I would hit a rough patch. The icing on the one-year cake was that we had recently upgraded from a three-bedroom condominium to a five-bedroom house.

That was when, two months later, we got a surprise: I was pregnant again. Once the shock of an unexpected pregnancy—and one with a fourteen-month-old underfoot—wore off, I really leaned in to the pregnancy. I was enthusiastic (a late summer arrival!) and hopeful (perhaps we'd get a boy!) and confident. After all, I had carried my daughter to term, so surely my past miscarriages were just that—a part of my medical history. It was almost as if I presumed that growing and birthing a baby had hit reset on my uterus. Then there were the words that never crossed my lips but floated in and out of my thoughts: this was my second chance at motherhood and—this time—I might get to do it without the black veil of postpartum depression.

By Thanksgiving I learned I had been overconfident. I miscarried that holiday weekend. This time, though, my body did the work for me, expelling what I could no longer have (whereas the previous two times had required surgery). I called my doctor from the bathroom, blood in sight, and she reminded me that there was nothing I could do. She told me that the next day—if I wanted—I could go to the hospital lab and have blood drawn to check my HCG levels to confirm my miscarriage.

I really didn't need confirmation, but I like data (it soothes me), and this would be data. (I am also typically a rule follower, and I knew from past experience that I'd have to get blood drawn at some point anyway.) So the following day I went to the hospital lab. But they didn't have an order from my doctor for any blood work to be drawn. They kindly called her, but a colleague of hers was now on call, and this doctor knew nothing about my change in status. I stood in the lab waiting room, using the technician's landline, while other patients sitting nearby listened in, and recounted the previous night's events. And once this doctor was up to speed (along with all the lab personnel and the waiting patients) she finally agreed to order a blood draw. As I sat in that cold vinyl chair and they wrapped a rubber tourniquet around my bicep, I silently cried.

Losing that baby rattled me emotionally nearly as much as the first miscarriage had. And my fear of being unsuccessful in having another viable pregnancy reached an all-time high. That fear was then channeled into finding answers.

Was there a common theme to my miscarriages?

Could I do anything to help make those babies "stick"?

Was there something I *shouldn't* do?

My fact-finding, answer-seeking interests led me back to my OBGYN. But I didn't like her answers, so I turned to the other physicians in the practice. Their responses were nothing short of consistent: from what they told me, they do not explore a potential cause for spontaneous pregnancy loss until you have experienced three miscarriages in a row. Not three total but three in a row. My daughter's birth, as it turns out, did reset something: the clock on getting answers.

A few months later, I interviewed another doctor at a different practice. I wasn't now exploring the idea of another provider solely because my current practice wouldn't go down the answer-seeking rabbit hole with me. If I'm being truly honest, yes, that did play a role, but also their approach had felt a little laissez-faire: I had heard from them that "it would happen" and that "sometimes it's not meant to be." That had cut me so deeply and left me feeling unheard and unseen. And so I looked elsewhere and fortunately almost immediately met the OBGYN I needed: Dr. Kim. She listened and empathized with me and my husband and soothed us and agreed to not only accompany me on my fact-finding mission but also lead us.

With her as our guide, I starting checking off tests and eliminating potential causes. A few months later, still answerless, I was pregnant for the fifth time.

And then I miscarried.

But the defeat felt different this time. It was softer and mellower. I also had a road map to keep following—and that kept me feeling hopeful. It was as if Dr. Kim bled and sweated empathy. She handled me gently, and it was exactly what I needed.

Equally important, especially as I felt like I was getting closer to a viable pregnancy, is that we made a plan for after my delivery and how to tackle another potential bout of postpartum depression. I was, understandably, concerned. After my first daughter had been born, it had been my mother who'd noticed a shift in me; she was the one who'd driven me to my follow-up appointment and gently insisted that I talk to my then-OBGYN about my mental state. I hadn't been able to see it, and neither had my husband. And so now I needed Dr. Kim to understand how blind we'd been—and as someone who tends to lean toward proactivity in medical concerns versus reactivity, I wanted to outline early on what I could do before any baby arrived to head off postpartum depression at the pass.

I decided to take matters into my own hands partly because I was so often reminded of my postpartum depression at the most unexpected times—like when I applied for life insurance and my history of postpartum depression flagged me for a much higher rate. Though these were hard reminders of my past, a past that I had worked so hard to move beyond, they reinforced my need to make a comprehensive plan with Dr. Kim.

I continued with a few more tests, stopping short of the most invasive one. I'd cross that bridge if I needed to, but for now Dr. Kim and I had dialed in on a medication routine she felt confident would help me maintain a pregnancy, and we had a plan for monitoring my progress and medication needs if I were to conceive again. I also had a clear mental-health plan: as I neared the latter half of my third trimester, I would preemptively set up an appointment with my therapist for shortly after baby was born. And Dr. Kim and I would decide together before I was discharged from the hospital whether I would proactively start on an antidepressant or take a wait-and-see approach.

And then it happened again. I conceived! On November 18, 2014, my husband was, yet again, traveling overseas on business when I confirmed my sixth pregnancy and shared with him our good fortune by texting the picture of the positive pregnancy test. He responded warmly, and though I can't remember exactly what he said, I can vividly remember his asking, "Are you happy?" I also remember that this is when I snapped that smiling, teary-eyed bathroom selfie. I was over the moon.

The elation lasted until morning, and then fear set in. Would this one stick? Every trip to the bathroom was an opportunity to check on my pregnancy status. Going to the doctor to get my blood drawn became my security blanket. Every girls' night with my mom friends was my chance to ask all the crazy "I'm still pregnant, right?" questions I had swirling in my head.

Dr. Kim and her physician and nurse colleagues held my hand every step of the way, both literally and figuratively. As the weeks ticked by, my nausea set in, and I used this common pregnancy symptom as a way to ease my worry. The more nauseated I felt, the less scared I was. The green and sick feeling finally passed as I entered my third trimester. We knew we were expecting another baby girl, and she and I had been tested for nearly everything we could to confirm that she was healthy and developmentally typical. Aside from finishing her nursery, the only thing I had left to do was make an appointment with my therapist.

Our younger daughter arrived just shy of one month before her due date. Her birth was beautiful. It was love at first sight—again. And the things that I had felt were, for lack of a better word, missteps that I'd made in the early days after my first daughter's birth I made sure to avoid this second time around. My pediatrician recommended my baby receive a small bolus of formula initially because her blood sugar was low.

"Go for it," was my reply, as I was not in a rush to force breastfeeding; I knew it would come. Would I like for her to go to the nursery for a couple of hours so I could sleep between feedings?

"Yes, absolutely." This time I understood that sleep helped me regulate my emotions better. I didn't skip meals, being sure to make good nutrition a priority. I kept visitors to a minimum, but I did allow them—unlike that first time.

I really prioritized our health.

Some time within my daughter's first two weeks of life I was able to have an appointment with my therapist. I remember crying; I do not remember what we discussed, but the session provided me with an emotional outlet. I went back the next week and the week after that and so on, until she told me the news that I had been—perhaps unknowingly—holding my breath over: I did not have postpartum depression.

Nor was I showing signs of developing it. Hearing that wasn't as fulfilling as I'd thought it might be, but I suspect this is because deep down I'd already known I was okay this time. I like to attribute this to my proactivity, but I guess I'll never know.

Even without a mental-health diagnosis, this time around I made sure to continue to prioritize our combined mental and physical health. I coordinated and employed as much assistance as I could, and I kept up with my weekly therapy sessions for about five months postpartum. We parted ways for a second time about when I returned to work full time.

This is where I want the story to end.

But life doesn't always play out as we envision it.

In all of my worrying about whether I was okay, and checking in with myself to assess whether my PPD was going to rear its ugly head again,

I'd forgotten to check in on my marriage. It's like we'd recognized that going from a couple to a family after our older daughter arrived was this big, momentous shift, but then when daughter number two came along, we didn't acknowledge the shift to a family of four with that same serious weight. It *is* different, though, to go from playing two-on-one defense to one-on-one defense. There's a shortage of what feels like everything. Maybe because our younger daughter was healthy and I hadn't relapsed into postpartum depression, my husband and I didn't even acknowledge that we'd entered into a new normal. I honestly don't know—and I doubt I will *ever* truly know.

Although it's easy for me to see that somewhere in that first year of raising our younger daughter my husband and I got lost, I think that our relationship shift occurred, perhaps even more profoundly, after the birth of our first. It's common wisdom that children take a toll on a marriage, but it's common wisdom that very few people actually speak meaningfully, or honestly, about.

As we'd gotten our bearings raising two children, we'd carried on with the other parts of our lives—namely, our careers and social calendar—as if nothing had changed.

But things *had* changed. I think there was a part of me that deeply resented my husband's inability to recognize that I was struggling with postpartum depression in those early days. Though I can say, rationally, that I'd also found it hard to identify what was going on with me at the time, I wish he'd stepped in to help in the way that my mom had—or in any way at all. Not that he wasn't a hands-on father, but he hadn't seen me.

And in realizing this, I realized that, perhaps, he still wasn't really seeing me.

You know that saying, though: hindsight is twenty-twenty. Looking back, as the pressure of two full-time careers and raising two small children built, I became someone I didn't want to be. I wonder now whether this transformation was a version of postpartum depression or postpartum anxiety. I am not sure. I remember feeling more like myself but simultaneously never feeling fully at peace. Very little in our day-to-day lives met my high standards. I was easily irritated at home. I kept searching for things to improve—redecorate this part of the house, work toward a promotion at work, et cetera, et cetera, et cetera. In other words, I was leaning in to everything in my life that I could, all the while letting my self-care slip.

Not too long after my younger daughter's second birthday, I reached out to a woman who'd gone to my same high school but whom I didn't know. I'd graduated with her husband and through the magic of Facebook had come across her blog, where she chronicled her own journey with postpartum depression. I mustered up the courage to send her a private Facebook message, and I'm so glad I did. Though we live across the country from one another, we have been emotionally inseparable ever since.

Right after I first reached out to her, this woman—Rebecca Fox Starr—sent me the following quotation: "There is a kind of a sort of cost. And a couple of things get lost. There are bridges you crossed you didn't know you crossed until you've crossed."

With my younger daughter's fourth birthday now on the horizon, I can see which bridges I have crossed and when. I walked over Anxiety Ocean, I bootstrapped my way through Do-It-All-Yourself, I waded through Career-Enhancing Creek. When I finally stopped and looked around, I realized I'd traveled all that way alone. I'd journeyed solo to an emotional island. I tried to retrace my steps, but I couldn't fill in the ocean that had spread between my daughters' father, now my ex-husband, and me. As cliché as it sounds, not everything is fixable.

I never expected that this would be how my story would go, but I'm truly grateful that this is how it did. Because every step I took, every misstep I took, every hole I dug myself out of, and every mountain I summited made me who I am today. And I really like that person.

AMANDA, THIRTY-THREE YEARS OLD

As we stood at our wedding under the chuppah, a sacred Jewish canopy, the rabbi thought it would be funny and appropriate to bless us with the ability to have thirteen children. Everyone in attendance had a good laugh, and somewhere deep down inside both of our hearts, my husband and I knew that it would really be the dream, as unrealistic as it sounded. To our peers and mentors, who are orthodox Jews, it seemed less crazy to adhere to the strict Jewish laws as a guidebook in our everyday lives, including the injunction to *be fruitful and multiply*. Large families are expected in our community. But in all seriousness, to be fruitful and multiply is the first thing God commands Adam and Eve in the Book of Genesis—right from the start. And from the start of my journey with my husband, even when were just dating, we'd discussed how many children we'd want (six), what their names would be (our first boy would be Jonah), and even on what timeline (pop 'em out as fast as possible).

Living in an orthodox Jewish community can sometimes make newly-weds feel pressured to have children right away. It's that look you get from someone, a few months after you're married, that just *tells* you they're wondering whether you're pregnant yet. Or worse, when you've been married for "a while" and still haven't shown signs of fertility (not that it's anyone's business, right?). Many friends of ours decide to wait a year or more before even trying to get pregnant, attributable to various reasons: finishing school, building a financial nest, or buying a house. All too often, you learn of someone who's unable to get pregnant, and that's when you really start to remember that this type of information is no one's business but their own. But as for my husband and me? We simply needed time to get our ducks in a row, travel, and enjoy some time together before life would get crazy with kids.

As a result of our decision to wait a bit, we spent the first year of our marriage exploring some of the many issues we hadn't yet understood about each other, despite the eleven months we'd spent together leading up to our wedding day. But buying a home, building up a small savings, and working through all the newness had to come first. I was just about thirty years old then, and I figured that if I spent the vast majority of the next ten years producing and raising babies, we'd meet our goal to fill our house with kids before I was forty.

When the time finally came to start our family, getting pregnant didn't take long. After having been on birth control for a solid twelve years, I'd expected it to take a little while. But sure enough, two months after we started trying, we were on our way to baby number one. The pregnancy, in its entirety, was easy and smooth. I didn't take this for granted for even one day. My husband had no idea how easy he'd had it, though. A wife who didn't throw up constantly? No scary complications along the way? I'd never expected him to know what women talk about in close circles of friends regarding our bodies and the more bizarre parts of being pregnant, but I thanked God every day that *I wasn't* throwing up, that I didn't have gestational diabetes, and that I was even able to teach my weekly Zumba classes with ease up until the end of my third trimester.

When I went into labor on that late Saturday night in December 2017, I had what many would call a lucky experience, although it seemed traumatic to me in the moment. A *silent labor*, my doula called it. No symptoms of labor, although my body had been secretly progressing in disguise. At around 9:30 P.M., the contractions had hit so hard that I'd thought I would deliver my baby in the toilet at home—or maybe I'd even die. One of the two options seemed imminent. It was as if my completely peaceful pregnancy had been a trick—only the period of calm before the turbulent storm.

The night I went into labor I'd watched a movie and then gone to take a hot shower, and the next thing I knew, I was screaming for my husband because I couldn't stand up or get back into my clothes. I was having one long, never-ending contraction. It was soon confirmed at the hospital that the immense pain was because I was already dilated seven centimeters. What about laboring at home? What about feeling the contractions get closer together over time? And what about that stupid blue yoga ball I hadn't even yet used but bought for this very moment? I got an epidural immediately, pushed for a few hours, and before the sun came up, we welcomed into the world our daughter, Zahava.

The two months of maternity leave that followed pretty much felt, for this workaholic, like the equivalent of quitting my job for a year. I was barely able to stay off my e-mail because I so badly wanted to keep myself in the loop and know what I was missing there. It was a newer job for me—one I was committed to and sad to be away from. I really didn't understand what maternity leave was meant for, and before I knew it, I was getting ready to go back to work, eight weeks later.

And so that first week of February I jumped back into work so fast that it's only in retrospect I understand how little I'd appreciated the time off with my newborn baby girl. I'd spent those two quick months on leave going to Target, getting coffee with friends, visiting family in New York, and binge-watching *Gilmore Girls*. I hadn't understood the magnitude of exhaustion that would hit me eight quick weeks postpartum upon return to work.

From the moment I went back to work, I wasn't sure what was worse: schlepping my daughter every morning to the nanny, being at work while the messes in my house accumulated, or constantly fighting with my husband about things so unimportant that I can't even remember them to describe here. I just blamed the hormones for everything (as did my husband), though it hadn't quite occurred to me that something deeper, something chemical, and something *real* was brewing inside my brain.

So there I was, standing in my closet trying to get dressed for work, crying. In fact, I wasn't just crying, I was bawling, and I had no clue why.

Why was my husband upsetting me about everything imaginable? Why didn't any of my clothes fit me yet? Why was I always late for work now when I've been punctual my whole life? Why was my brain totally messing with me when I'm one of the most level-headed and realistic people I know? I understood this to be part of motherhood and parenthood; I didn't think it was something that could be diagnosed.

"Call your doctor *today*," my mom said. She knew something sounded off in my tone of voice when I was explaining to her how yet again today I'd stood in my underwear, crying in my closet, while my husband angered me about things I couldn't even relay to her. I'd made it to work and had been sitting at a colleague's desk, doing the morning catch-up, when my mom had called to say hello. I hadn't told any friends at work how miserable I'd been feeling, but after hearing my mom's concern, I excused myself to go call my doctor.

"Yes, I was fine at my six-week appointment," I explained to the receptionist, "but now I'm almost nine weeks postpartum, and I need to be seen again."

"What are your symptoms?" She evidently felt it was her job to get a full-panel explanation of what I was going through in order to book the appointment.

"I'm at work, and I'm not about to discuss the details, but I know I need to be seen by the doctor as soon as possible," I politely pushed. She found a slot that day at 2:00 P.M. I'd be there.

My doctor asked me a slew of questions that seemed pretty routine for the average crazy, postpartum, new mom. She confirmed that all of my symptoms were pretty normal, and if I wanted to consider medication to balance things out, she told me she'd fill a prescription that day for a common, low-dosage mood stabilizer. By that time I was no longer nursing my daughter, and it seemed pretty obvious that I'd have to surrender to the medication if I wanted to feel sane again. I don't recall my doctor actually telling me I was being diagnosed with postpartum depression. I just knew I needed some temporary help getting my life back together. I'd always been on top of my game, punctual and precise, hardworking, and, at times, a perfectionist. I had been beating myself up to try and still be that person, unaware that my life had shifted so much as a mother and that nothing would ever be the same again.

I'd never taken medication for depression or anxiety in my entire life, although I'd probably been a candidate for it during high school, college, and throughout my twenties. I'd had my fair share of dysfunctional-family problems, daddy issues, self-identity searches, bad breakups, and so on. But this was real, married-with-kids type of stuff. Something felt much more heavy about this turmoil, and I just wanted to *feel normal* again. When I said yes to my doctor and to that prescription that day, I felt as if I'd signed myself up for something vaguely shameful.

I'd always felt I could work through my issues naturally and be strong enough to say I didn't need help to do what I needed to do. And so I was ashamed that I was giving in to prescription meds. I was ashamed I couldn't deal with it on my own, unmedicated. It felt dishonest to be "okay" by way of drugs. I felt like I would be lying to the world around me to slap a smile on my face only because the meds were making me. But maybe, I thought, I really did have a chemical imbalance that was fighting my true ability to be happy again. Maybe I was *irrationally* angry at my husband, lashing out at him day and night. Perhaps I hadn't been as ready to return to work as I'd thought.

And so I filled the prescription and started taking the meds. It felt miraculous. Within a day or two I felt better—as if those the little blue pills kicked in as fast as I had gotten pregnant. I didn't cry for a few days straight, which was amazing considering where I'd been coming from. I just couldn't believe what I was experiencing. It started to make me feel more justified and validated in my decision to medicate. As I began opening up to a few friends about what I was doing to help manage my life and my emotional distress, I realized that so many people, right here in my own neighborhood, and even within my circle of friends, were just like me. So if this thing I was suffering from was so common, was it really, technically, postpartum depression? Or was it just par for the course? Everything up until now had been such a blur. Did I have something diagnosable, or were my postpartum experiences "normal," as the doctor had said they were? Was I a *victim* of PPD, or was I a *survivor*? The questions ran through my head. If it was real, if I really had PPD, then I'd really gone through something heavy. And that seemed really significant.

Within a couple months of feeling much better about life in general, my husband and I concluded that I felt "fine enough" to have another baby. That had been the plan all along, right? We were also blessed with a first child that made motherhood seem far too simple. She slept on schedule, ate on schedule, allowed *me* to sleep and eat on schedule . . . I was pretty sure that this wasn't the norm for most new mothers and that I was lucky. And if I'd been lucky once, maybe I had a good shot at being lucky again. The decision wasn't too well thought out, and everything happened so fast. We sort of just went with the program and left it up to fate (and a packet of ovulation test strips).

On Saturday afternoon of my first Mother's Day weekend, I suffered a case of heartburn so severe it jolted me awake. I'd been taking a nap next to my husband, when I suddenly woke up to a terrible, burning pain behind my breastbone. I nudged him awake and told him how badly it hurt. He opened bleary eyes and mumbled "You're pregnant" before shutting his eyes and rolling over, back into oblivion. I couldn't believe what he'd just said. Pregnant? But was it possible?

I suppose it was *possible*: after having decided that it was maybe time to start on baby number two, we hadn't been as careful with our birth control, and there was that *one time* . . .

But on a scale of one to highly unrealistic, I assumed that pregnancy wasn't likely.

Later that night I took a pregnancy test, which confirmed exactly what my husband had predicted. And then I took two more pregnancy tests to confirm the first pregnancy test. They both came back positive. It had to be a scary joke. Part of me was happy, laughing inside, and part of me was in complete disbelief. Again—the plan—it was what we'd always imagined. But simultaneously I started envisioning depleted bank account balances, toy room messes, private school tuition . . . I lit a candle, hopped in the shower, and took a deep breath.

I knew my husband would be excited about the news. As for me, I was undecided. Everything seemed to be calm and okay since my recent decision to medicate. But the doctors had told me it could take up to a year after my daughter's birth for my body to fully heal. Would I be okay jumping back into pregnancy only five months after she'd been born? Would I have to stop taking the medication for the unborn baby's sake? Would this pregnancy be as easy as my last? Would I be able to keep teaching Zumba? *How on earth would I tell my job I had to go on maternity leave again—and this time possibly even longer if I wanted to take the full three months I was allowed to take?*

I wanted to be happy about this "on-purpose accident," but something inside me was unsure of the timing. I questioned my decision to have another baby even though I realized the decision had already been made. I started to question my ability to love more than one baby. I questioned how I would maintain my sanity and mental health if I went off medication in the upcoming months.

Alas, my first Mother's Day weekend would never be forgotten. Yes, I celebrated the joy of being a first-time mother, and even the joy of doing it again so very soon. But this also meant "celebrating" many other realities: I wouldn't be able to wear or buy any normal-sized clothes for another year or so. I would have to dig out my maternity clothes that I'd only just packed away. I'd also have to come to terms with caring for a newborn while chasing a one-year-old around the house. My kids would be a mere year and one month apart.

What I was not prepared for was for the next six to seven months to be asked at least once a day whether "this pregnancy was planned" and "how far apart my children were going to be." To say it was irritating would be an understatement. It was a constant reminder of the stress and difficulty that already came with balancing my life with one child and how it would only be compounded with this pregnancy and then my second child.

We made it through the summer, savoring each moment with our baby girl before her brother arrived months later. Depressed as I was to look at myself in the mirror—a postpartum body that wouldn't have a chance to go back to normal any time soon—I trudged through my days with the help of Zoloft and was happy to learn that it would be entirely safe for me to keep taking it throughout the entire pregnancy. I didn't ask whether I still needed it; I just knew that taking it kept so many issues at bay and that I wasn't yet willing to take the risk of trying to cope without it. Once or twice I'd forgotten my bedtime dose, and sure enough, within twenty-four hours my husband and I would be at war over something nonsensical. Those fights always came down to that one thing: that I'd forgotten my medication the night before. So I surrendered to the fact that the medication was still working and that taking it was still worth it.

At the end of the second trimester, on the eve of Sukkoth, a major Jewish holiday, I was cooking and cleaning, preparing for what should have been a fantastic few days with family and friends, when I picked up Zahava to put her in her high chair, and my back went out. This was no mere muscle strain. This was full force and far worse than any of the other times I'd had back problems pre- and postpregnancy. The pain rendered me immobile. I could not walk, I could not sit, I could not finish the cooking or the cleaning. I laid my pregnant self flat out on the bed and spent the next ten or so days horizontal. I worked from home for much of that time. Given the long list of medications contraindicated in pregnancy, I could take nothing to control my pain, which didn't subside, and I half cursed myself for having gotten into this mess in the first place. What kind of person lets themselves get pregnant so quickly without first making sure their body is strong and healthy enough beforehand? Me. I was that kind of person, and I wasn't happy about it. I pointed a finger at myself and fell back into my self-recriminating misery.

Physiatrists, spine surgeons, physical therapists . . . over those next excruciating weeks I saw them all. The results were inconclusive because no one would do an MRI on a pregnant woman in her second trimester. The rationale was that if they found something that warranted surgery, they couldn't do it anyway because of the baby, which meant they couldn't justify placing the baby at risk by performing the test in the first place. I walked around feeling misunderstood and in pain 24-7. At least physical therapy was (slowly) but surely mending my crookedness. I mean, I was *actually* crooked for two months.

A lot of assumptions were made about what was wrong with my sacroiliac joint and whether I'd potentially slipped a disc, but it didn't matter. I was in pain day and night for months straight. I could not lift my baby out of her crib or into her high chair. I could neither sit nor stand for more than fifteen minutes at a time without needing a full-body stretch. I could not go for a pedicure to treat myself or for a prenatal massage to reduce the stress of my busy work season. I was in too much pain and felt deeply sad all the time.

At work I was tired of colleagues jokingly telling me that I was still crooked, day after day, and eventually week after week. As if I were unaware of how I appeared. As if I could ignore the pain I felt at all times of day. I didn't want special accommodations; I didn't want to be helped to carry something to my office. I just wanted to go back to being the independent person I'd always had been, free of pain—and free from pregnancy. I wanted a do-over in my marriage, my family, and, ultimately, my life.

It was in my third trimester that I really began regretting and resenting my pregnancy. I hated who I'd become—feeling full of negativity at all times. I was teetering on two years straight of pregnancy and going on a year of PPD. I wanted them both to be over. I also wanted to stop going to doctors every week, I wanted to return to teaching Zumba classes without fearing the pain I'd be in the next day, and I wanted to wear the clothes in my closet that I hadn't been able to fit for so long.

The resentment permeated into everything I did and ultimately led me down a very negative path of foul language and thoughts toward everyone I knew. I couldn't find happiness in anything; I felt useless, unable to help lift an Amazon box from the doorway or put my daughter in her crib at bedtime. I had no energy left by the evening and certainly no energy first thing in the morning after a sleepless night of tossing and turning, unable to find comfort in any sleeping position. I cried myself to sleep night after night as my husband snored within moments of hitting the pillow. I felt alone, and I missed my old self.

My husband felt neglected, and I was angry to hear about it, knowing I could not change our situation. Faking an emotional connection to another human being was just not an option at this my all-time low. I would often tell him it wasn't my fault we couldn't be intimate, but at the same time I also blamed myself for maybe not trying hard enough to care about his feelings and needs. I was simply in too much discomfort and felt too depressed to let my mind go anywhere beyond the daily tasks necessary to running a household and being a mother. I was lucky I could even do that. But thankfully, with the help of my mother and mother-in-law, I got through each day. They understood my pain, they understood my struggle as a new mom, and they understood my inner conflict over wanting to grow my family while also wanting to get out of this personal hell.

About a month or so before Jonah was born, I quietly took myself off the Zoloft. I mentioned it to my doctor, saying I was just experimenting to see how I would do. As backward as it may sound now, I thought that if I went off the medication, maybe my sex drive would come back and my husband and I would miraculously fix our marriage just in time for our son to be born. But my problems ran much deeper than a low sex drive. My days and nights were filled with counting down the minutes until my son would be born so I could immediately begin to rebuild myself and my strength. In any case, my doctor said it was a perfectly fine for me to take myself off Zoloft—whatever the reasons. My back was now almost straight again, and the busyness of preparing for our son's imminent arrival overshadowed any symptoms of PPD craziness I'd once had. I wanted to test the waters and see if I could pull it off. I did not want these drugs in my system when the baby was born and I began nursing, hopefully, again.

Just as his sister had been, Jonah was born right on time at forty-one weeks late. This time, however, the signs of labor had been more obvious, and my birthing story was beautiful, calm, and quick. It was a perfect ending to a pretty miserable journey. I felt like I deserved this happy outcome, a sort of consolation prize for the amount of pain and inner conflict I'd been going through all the months of my pregnancy. The few days I spent in the hospital were like a mini-getaway—a vacation, if you will. I could finally be alone in the stillness and quiet with my baby.

But the entire time I was recovering in the maternity ward, I fiercely missed my daughter. I was trying so hard to bond with my new baby in so many ways (breastfeeding, taking photos, staring at him for hours on end as he slept), but I couldn't help but wonder what my little girl was doing at all times of the day. What was she eating? How was she napping? And did she even realize I was gone? I continued to beat myself up—and still do even as I write these words—for the distance I've placed between us by bringing her brother into the world. I must remind myself daily that this is the consequence of building a family, of doing it at a safe stage and age in my life, and that I can't reverse the situation I've created for myself.

Even today, almost six weeks later, I still miss her even when we're together. I can't hold a newborn and also hold her. It makes me sad when I hear her wake up in the morning, sometimes crying from the pain of teething, and I cannot be the hero that comforts her. Thankfully, my husband is a Number-One Father, and she adores him too. But as a mommy, I feel like I'm neglecting her and often doubt if more children could even be emotionally possible for me.

Within a few days of Jonah's birth, my husband asked me when we could have another baby. I nearly died just hearing him ask me that. He was so thankful for another healthy, beautiful baby and just wanted as many as possible. To be frank, at the time he asked me this, I hadn't even managed to go to the bathroom without pain since the labor. So there was no way we were discussing getting pregnant again at that point. If there is one way to start a fight with your wife while her hormones are at an all-time high, it would be by introducing this conversation. Through my tears, I explained that, although I, too, had once wanted a large family, I wasn't sure I could do this again. I told him that although I, too, had once expected to have babies all throughout my thirties, we had scored big time by getting a baby of each gender, and now we should possibly reconsider our plans. He felt like I was squashing his life dream, and I felt like he was squashing *me*. Unable to communicate healthily, we made an agreement to table the conversation until I was more emotionally stable and ready to talk about it, which he respected.

Today I'm nearly six weeks postpartum, and I haven't resorted to taking those small blue pills yet. I've had truly terrible nights of sleep deprivation as Jonah's fought to find his sleep rhythm, and I now see that there is a reason they call it *beginner's luck*. I don't remember being this tired or frazzled after my daughter's birth. I'm renavigating the breastfeeding experience and trying to figure out how to be alone with two babies while one is attached to my boob and one is learning to open every cabinet in the house. I have to constantly ask myself whether this is really what I wanted when I'd said I wanted a big family, and to create it at lightning speed.

More than anything, I want to be that woman who is still at the top of her game, who can be punctual and precise, hardworking both in my job and in my family life, and strive for perfection at all possible times. I know it's not entirely realistic, but it's who I am. The meds made me feel like I could handle it all and made me feel as close to my old myself as I'd felt in a long time. But for now, it would be enough to be able to hold my pee in when I sneeze or laugh and average five hours of sleep a night. I genuinely want to be a great mother and an amazing wife. I want to be the person I promised my husband I would be when we stood under the wedding canopy in 2015. I want to show up for him, for Zahava, and for Jonah, and do whatever I have to do to stay healthy and happy. And I want to overcome the shame I felt last time I did what was necessary to stay happy and healthy.

And last but not least, I want to come to terms with knowing there's a chance we'll stay a family of four forever.

NIKKI, THIRTY YEARS OLD

I am a mother, and I am so much more. I am a survivor of perinatal mood and anxiety disorders. I am grateful for all my life experiences, for I now know my pain has a purpose. My story continues to grow every day, and that gives me a sense of peace and deep meaning.

My journey began in 2012 when my husband and I decided to start trying for a family. It did not come as easily as we'd expected, and so we had to endure infertility testing and eventually several cycles of infertility treatments. As a perfectionist, I found this very difficult; I felt like a failure for struggling to attain something I'd always planned for in my life. We ended up getting pregnant naturally after trying for eighteen months to conceive. Joy and relief.

I had a healthy pregnancy but was eventually put on bed rest for the last four weeks. Five days after my estimated due date, I delivered our healthy baby boy. He made his grand arrival during the Atlanta "Snowpocalypse," otherwise known as the blizzard of 2014. It was a long, intense labor and delivery with many moments of uncertainty, but even as harrowing as that experience was, I couldn't know that the main trauma was yet to come.

The day after my son's birth, there was a miscommunication between the members of the hospital staff and me regarding the baby's security bands and the safety system. As a sleep-deprived, hormonal new mom, what I'd taken from the quick encounter was that my son was in grave danger. Though I was so upset that I'd become hysterical from this episode, I was dismissed by all. This was the start of my journey with constant, debilitating anxiety and panic, occurring particularly whenever I was separated from my son for any length of time or distance. It would be years before this trauma would eventually be diagnosed and treated by a professional.

After our son was born, my husband and I decided that since it'd taken so long to get pregnant the first time, we wouldn't actively work to prevent pregnancy, and, once again, it took us fifteen months of trying before we were successful, naturally, again.

In the summer of 2015, we found out that we were due the following March with our second little boy. This pregnancy was physically torturous for me. I was diagnosed with hyperemesis gravidarum—an extreme form of the nausea and vomiting people often refer to as "morning sickness"— and even had to be hospitalized several times. To help with my condition, I eventually was given a Zofran stomach pump, which was meant to abate my nausea and vomiting. Though the hospital stays were physically trying, the hardest part of it all was being separated—for the first time since his birth—from my nursing toddler.

Our second son surprised us by making a quick entrance into the world, two weeks ahead of schedule. His birth was honestly a breeze compared to my first experience, but that ease was very short-lived. I requested and was granted early release from the hospital. The familiar darkness of perinatal distress hit the moment we got home. I remember it so vividly: I felt crushed by the reality and pressure to now care for two little humans.

The overwhelming feeling sunk my heart and spirits. Again I hid my feelings and tried to be the "super mom" I'd thought I would always be. I'm a perfectionist, which makes it so hard for me to admit to of my perceived weaknesses. I'd always thought that my desire to be a mother would mean that I would feel like an amazing mother. That I would be happy and grateful. The expectations did not match the reality. When our new addition was just eighteen days old, our family suffered a devastating loss: my father-in-law died by suicide. This was a crushing blow, come at a time when emotions were already running high, and so I began to feel, now more than ever, the need to be strong for everyone else. There was no way I could ask for help when everyone around me was grieving.

Once again, I did not ask for help, and so help I did not get.

I struggled every single day, never once speaking up and asking for support. At that point, in the midst of my suffering, it was obvious to me that I was done having kids. I could not endure the pain again, and so I began using birth control right away. I hit rock bottom in 2017, a year after our second son's birth, and knew that without help I would not survive another year. So I resigned myself to make a change. I started taking an antidepressant and sought therapy in January 2018. My recovery was slow and took patience. The psychological underpinnings to my condition became interesting to me, and so I pursued mental-health training and events to aid in my healing. I even started my own local and online peer-support group.

It was not until the summer of that year when something in me shifted and I started to even entertain the idea of having another child. My boys were now four and two, the oldest about to head off to pre-K in the fall. Life had finally settled down, and I was feeling in control and happy for the first time in a long time. I was looking at life through a new lens. Together, my partner and I made the decision to stop using birth control. I was anxious but at the same time felt at ease for many reasons.

Knowledge is power, and that I now possessed. I was now armed with information on risk factors for perinatal mood and anxiety disorders, their symptoms, their treatment, and so much more. I now had a support system, and I knew how to ask for help. I was confident that my newfound awareness and psychoeducation would be an added layer of protection to guard my mental health in the future.

A major reason why I now felt comfortable expanding our family was the support plan we had in place. I'd decided that, should I become pregnant, I would continue to stay on my medication for the entire pregnancy and throughout the postpartum period. I knew with confidence that in my case the benefits outweighed the risks.

My local family would also be available and be encouraging of my self-care time. They would provide practical help and babysitting weekly to ensure that I'd have adequate time to sleep, eat, and exercise.

As fate would have it, we got pregnant immediately. For the first time we were expecting with quick success. I write this as I am pregnant, and now due in May 2019 with baby number three. We will be surprised by the gender, but in all other ways we have things covered. While I have been having a hard time again physically this pregnancy, I have been feeling healthy mentally. This feels like a huge accomplishment. I am hopeful about my birth and postpartum experience because of the knowledge I have attained and plans I have set in place to protect my mental health. I am proud to say that I am a mother and so much more. I am a survivor! I made my way into the light, and I am committed to helping other moms join me there.

5

❖ ❖

24-7, 365: Adoption After Postpartum Depression

It was the first cold Sunday of the season. It was October. Hundreds of tiny Legos were splayed out on the basement rug before me, as my son clicked them together in intricate shapes and patterns, giving voices to his creations as he built, happily. He is such a content child.

He and I were home alone together for the afternoon. We hunkered down in our basement, lying down on the plush carpet, savoring the warmth of the cozy room, of each other's presence. Just before our play-time together, he had let me hold him in my arms to cradle him, and he asked me for "one hundred kisses." I kissed his face, slowly and deliberately, lingering on his chin. His chin was the first thing I had noticed about him when they'd placed his head next to mine in the operating room on a different cold October afternoon five years prior. The prominent dimple in his chin is something that I have loved about him, intensely, for his entire life, even when it was hard to love much of anything.

I listened to my son's sweet little timbre as he played a game with his Legos called Spider-Man versus Stingman, creating distinct voices for each of his characters.

I did not want to interrupt him, but I was having a hard time containing myself. I felt so filled up. That familiar, uncomfortable, big feeling was bubbling up inside of me, and I figured he was the best human in whom I could confide.

I wrestled with the worry that I might be burdening him, but I could not control myself.

"Hey, buddy?" I asked—interrupting a particularly snarky bit of dialogue, in which Stingman asked, "Why would I be your friend?" before zapping his foe.

"Zzzzzzzzz," Beau buzzed, before turning to me, signaling that he was giving me a moment of his attention.

I looked at his eyes, blue and wide and shiny, like icy marbles.

"You know how I had my two babies?" I continued.

"And then they grew up into kids, right?" he completed the thought. He really hammered that point home, for me.

"Right. And I don't have any other babies now . . ." I trailed off.

I wanted to ask him what to do next. I wanted for him to build me an answer out of Legos because he's so good at Legos. Sometimes the thoughts in my head are so chaotic that they actually resemble the giant mess of Legos on the basement floor, all in different shapes and colors, some stuck together and some alone, abandoned.

With the Legos, even when the mess feels enormous, there's always a clear—albeit tedious and laborious—way to clean it up. I wanted for Beau to build me a bridge. I longed for him to build me a connection from me to the other baby that is in my heart, big enough and strong enough to cross the moat and to ward off the dangerous creatures below.

And if he could not do that, I wanted him to ask me for a baby. Truthfully, I wanted him to beg me for a baby. If Beau begged me for a new, little sibling, then the decision would be easier, I told myself, trying desperately to believe my own story. The sacrifices and risks would seem less selfish, as I would be giving him the gift that I'd given Belle when I'd given birth to him. There are so many things that, because of my postpartum depression, I was unable to give to him, and I think I will forever want to make this up to him. And at the same time, I realized that wanting him to ask me for something so that I could feel less selfish about wanting it is a supremely selfish notion in itself.

Instead of listening to my wise mind, I gave into its weaker counterpart. I could be more kind to myself and call it my *emotional* mind, but sometimes they feel like the same thing.

"So, would you *want* another baby?"

"Yes. I want a baby. In the pink room!"

"You'd put the baby in the pink room?" I asked, referring to our extra bedroom, directly next to his own. Knowing (believing) that I would not have another baby for whom we would need the bedroom, I had painted it in a color that I liked—a soft pink, with metallic gold doors—and have used it as an upstairs play area for the kids.

"I wouldn't put it there; that would just be the baby's room." He was cool in his speech, looking away from me to put a tiny, plastic flame into the hands of his miniature hero.

I started to cry, silently. Because I did not want him to see me crying, I did not ask him whether I could join in his game; rather, I pivoted, keeping my face hidden from his view. I started to clean up the Lego mess, as I tried to sort through the chaos in my head. Tears fell onto the tiny, colored blocks, and with every handful I picked up, the pieces seemed to multiply. I started to paw at the toys with both hands, putting them into plastic bins haphazardly, grabbing them so frantically, without being mindful of their sharp edges, that my hands began to hurt.

As the tears continued to fall, and as my hands grew sore, I looked up at my son. My blue-eyed boy, creative and strong and determined boy. My Beau.

I looked at his chin, and my heart fell into my stomach, in a way that was both good and hard at the same time.

"Maybe this is enough," I mouthed noiselessly to myself, as I picked up another handful of Legos, threw them into the plastic bin, and wiped my nose on my sweater.

It was the first cold Sunday of the season. It was October. I was battling with Legos, willing them to give me the answers. Longing for control. Putting away the pieces.

"Mommy," Beau came up behind me. "There are still some more Legos on the floor."

"It's okay," I told him, squeaking out the words as I choked on my tears.

Because even though I'd tried so hard to hide it, he'd managed to uncover my secret. He just didn't know what it was he'd uncovered—that I was leaving just enough of the pieces out in front of me so that maybe, someday, I would figure out a way to build a drawbridge so that I could safely cross the moat.

For Kenny and me, adoption has always seemed like a really meaningful way to expand our family. Giving a child a home feels like the greatest gift that we could both give and receive. For a long time after we'd begun the discussion of expanding our family in our post-postpartum-depression-reality, adoption had been Kenny's preferred method of family expansion. He'd felt strongly that it would be the right decision for us, as it would be "doing a mitzvah," as he says, and, as I am keenly aware, it would take some of his greatest fears off the table.

We do not look at adoption as a consolation prize, second choice, or backup plan. We also do not judge those who do feel as though adoption is a backup plan. It makes sense; we know many couples who have tried for years to have a baby biologically and then, when it became clear to them that, for one reason or another, they could not, grew a baby in their hearts as opposed to their wombs. It is beautiful to behold.

As with everything, the notion of adoption is quite different in theory than it is in practice. The grand ideas that I have had swirling in my head were colorful and, at times, magical, but they would not just manifest on their own. Taking the first step toward the adoption process meant educating myself, both with literature and, more important, with real-life information. I first decided to take this leap at the end of 2017, between my first and second rounds of IVF.

I sent a text message to a woman I know who works as a caseworker for a local adoption agency. My message was long, and it was rambling, and it was emotional, enough so that she suggested we speak on the phone. I can remember dialing her number from the quiet of my basement and that my heart was racing as I spoke. For some reason, I felt the need to explain myself and why I was coming to her for information about adoption when, for so many years prior, I had been lamenting the fact that I could no longer have children. Despite our personal relationship, she remained professional and measured, and she gave me a high-level overview of the adoption process. She gave me the name of another local caseworker and suggested we attend a group meeting that would be taking place the following month.

I did not attend the meeting, however. I do not remember exactly what had come up, and perhaps it's because we decided to try for that next round of IVF, but the bottom line is that I think I chickened out. It was months later when I finally called the woman whose number my friend had given me and explained our situation to her. I told her that, while we have the ability to have a baby biologically, and while we do have two children already, we do not feel complete. I told her that adoption has always felt like a good option for us. In my head, I can remember thinking, "It feels noble, and it feels right, but I need to make sure that the latter outweighs the former."

The kind caseworker further allayed my worries about being an "atypical case" by explaining that while we did not fit the average profile for new, adoptive parents, we had a lot of attributes in our favor. First, for an adoptive mother, we could show a proven track record of having raised two happy, great kids. She explained that many adoptive mothers would want to know that their baby would be going into a home that was not just loving but also filled with cheerful noise, like siblings, pets, and family-friendly activity. Typically, she explained, an adoptive mother does not want to think of her baby as being someone's last choice. In our case, it would be abundantly clear that we were adopting because we *wanted* to and not because we *had* to.

I learned that there are many kinds of adoptions and that Kenny and I would have to make some big decisions—and that some big decisions would be made for us. I had heard enough about adoption to know that there was foreign adoption (when you adopt a child from another country) and also domestic adoption (when you adopt a child from the United States). I also knew, loosely, about open adoptions and closed adoptions and that there were options in the middle, but I wasn't quite sure what those were. It was my understanding that with open adoptions the birth mother would choose the adoptive parents, the adoptive parents would know the identity of the birth mother, and, presumably, they could all continue to have an ongoing relationship throughout the child's life. I thought that a closed adoption was when the birth parents and adoptive parents had minimal contact, if at all, and that the child would not have any with the birth parents. I had absolutely no idea what options existed in the middle; I just knew they were out there.

My talks with the caseworkers from the adoption agency were informative and, to be truthful, more than just a little bit overwhelming. But, I reminded myself, if adoption was the right choice for our family, calling the adoption agencies would be the easiest step. I would have to buck up and be just as forceful and fastidious and thorough in my investigation of this option as I had been in my medical research surrounding a potential future pregnancy. And there was also one question that I could not avoid asking, try as I might:

Would an adoption agency allow me to adopt a child knowing that I have suffered from mental illness? And if so, would any potential birth mother even want me?

The agencies I spoke to were compassionate and, once again, assured me that, while I would have to get documentation from my psychologist, stating that I was mentally fit, I was already an established mother, and a good one at that. I am supremely grateful that adoption agencies are so thorough in their background checks. I wouldn't want to have it any other way. It is an ironic, and somewhat dark, notion, but this is one of the only situations in which I am treated the same way as someone who has suffered from a physical disease. Besides qualifying for health insurance and life insurance, the mentally ill and the physically ill (or, in this case, the formerly mentally ill and the formerly physically ill) are not often lumped together or placed in the same category. Now, like anyone else who has been sick in ways measurable and immeasurable, I am a person who needs the adult equivalent of a permission slip in order to make a big life decision—in order to even be considered.

The next step of my journey was to talk to other humans. Before Beau, I had worked as a teacher for many years. Though I had originally planned to teach high school English, upon having Belle, I focused my career on music and early childhood education. Because many of my classes had been designed for parents and their young children to attend together, I'd gotten to know my fair share of families who have been formed, or fortified, through adoption. I spoke, casually, to several mothers who had gone through the adoption process in order to become parents, and their stories inspired me. Seeing the love these moms had for their children helped to assuage my fears that our third child might feel "less than" because he or she would not share our DNA.

I sought out adoptive mothers for their advice, deliberately, and then, on one occasion, an opportunity was gifted for me, and it took me by surprise. Fortuitously, I was given the chance to speak to a woman whom I respect tremendously who was actively going through the adoption process. It came up in conversation, and when I apologized for potentially prying, she assured me that she's an "open book." Speaking to someone in the thick of the adoption process was so helpful and so meaningful. This woman has two children, both considerably older than her third child would be. She'd checked in with them numerous times to make sure they felt comfortable with the notion of adding a new baby to the family, and they were.

Our conversation was partly about logistics. I asked her for the name of her adoption agency, and she shared with me what kind of adoption they had chosen to pursue. She told me how her plans fit with her family's values, and she spoke so earnestly, and with so much love, and I was moved, deeply. She said that she would tell the baby his or her birth story from the moment they all drove home from the hospital together—that it would always be known, just like any other birth story. Adoption, she explained, is not just one, finite act. A child is not just "adopted" as if it is an event that occurred in the past tense. She explained that she would always tell her child that they were able to become a family through the process of adoption and that this is just their story, with neither secrets nor fanfare. I love this so much.

I began to feel confident that, as a nurturer, I would help my child know that we hadn't just wanted him or her as much as we wanted Belle and Beau but that we'd wanted him or her *so* much that we did everything in our power, and had to work much harder, to bring him or her home to us. It is not a more or less thing. You can want two things with equal amounts of desire, just in different ways.

In talking to the mothers and the caseworkers and the family members, however, I also learned of some of the hard parts of adoption. One mother, whose bright, happy daughter had been in one of my first early childhood classes, had suffered the devastating loss of a failed adoption. I did not pry, but from what I gleaned, she'd gone through the entire process, taken care of the birth mother, prepared her daughter and family for a new baby, traveled to the birth mother's home state for the baby's delivery, and come home without her new baby. This, to me, was a whole new flavor of devastation. It was also further support for my belief that it does not matter if your child grows in your uterus or in your heart—your child is your child.

When I am asked about expanding our family, I often get feelings of marked anxiety. It is such a charged topic, and one for which Kenny and I have no answers, and so it feels like being trapped on an elevator. An elevator that keeps moving, and I'm just along for the ride. The car, suspended by cables and pulleys, lifts us up and then brings us down, and I cannot get off. In reality, elevator rides give me vertigo. Figuratively, this ride makes me dizzy, all the same.

But for some reason, when I talk to people about adoption, a sense of peace washes over me. Perhaps it's because it feels less selfish, which may or may not be true. Perhaps it's because it feels less risky, which may or may not be true. Perhaps it's because I know that my family members and friends would worry about me less, which may or may not be true. Or perhaps it's because, deep in my heart, this is the option that feels right. If the elevator would only stop at the floor marked *Adoption*, then I would gladly get off, steady myself, and start the process. But, alas, it keeps on moving.

Knowledge is power, we are told, and I find the adage holds true in so many cases; in the case of expanding my family, especially in a way about which I had less knowledge than I could have imagined, the more I could learn, the better it would be for everyone involved. I ended up finding out that I had been right about some of the things I'd believed formerly about adoption, and in other cases I'd been so incredibly wrong.

I am glad that adoption is increasingly considered a viable and valuable option for family expansion in our country and across the world. But the information available about it is lacking or confusing (or both).

I had originally assumed, naively, that most adoptions would be closed. Of the people I've known who either have adopted or were adopted, their adoptions have been completely closed, with no information or interaction.

According to a 2012 article in the *Washington Times*, based on a study performed by the Donaldson Adoption Institute, only 5 percent of domestic adoptions of infants are closed adoptions.[1] When I relayed this information to Kenny, he was just as shocked as I had been. We had both naively imagined that the majority of adoptions were (what we had thought of as) closed adoptions, so we were incredibly surprised to learn that the overwhelming national trend has been toward open adoptions. We were eager to learn about the levels of openness in adoption and the research supporting this shift in practice.

As the Donaldson Adoption Institute study states, "55 percent of domestic infant adoptions are 'fully disclosed.' This means birth and adoptive families know each other and typically have ongoing, direct contact," and "another 40 percent of infant adoptions are 'mediated,' which means families exchange letters and pictures through intermediaries, but they do not know each other." The study goes on to explain that a mere 5 percent of the remaining infant adoptions in the United States are officially "closed," which means that they are confidential and the adoptive parents are given medical records and information about the baby's biological parents but are not given their names or any identifying information.[2]

In order to process this information, I needed to better understand these different types of adoption. That was the only way I would be able to create a proper mental picture of our potential future family—one that was not obscured or opaque.

And then, after years of searching for data on an actual, real-life person who had not solely adopted, or been adopted, but had chosen to adopt post-postpartum depression, I struck gold. Well, almost; I got close enough to marvel at its gleam without really being able to touch it. I first read Amy Brannan's story featured in a *Postpartum Progress* piece—"7 Postpartum Depression Survivors Share Their Stories of Having More Children."[3] Amy, who has her own blog, *Living Life Joyously*, describes herself as a survivor of postpartum depression and anxiety and the "mama to three beautiful children, all unique and special in their own way."[4] Though I made many efforts to contact Amy, I was never able to speak to her directly, but I became something of an Amy expert nonetheless. Amy started blogging in 2009, two years after her daughter was born and she'd subsequently been walloped with a serious case of postpartum depression. In scouring her archived posts, I found one published on June 10, 2010, titled "A First for Me Today," in which she says that she had just bought the first baby thing for a potential future baby.[5] The post is short—only three sentences—but in it she describes her mixed (and strong) emotions surrounding the notion of having another baby after all she had endured. Seven months later, Amy announced on her blog that she and her husband had posted their profile on an online site for birth mothers in the United States and that they were hoping to expand their family through adoption.[6] The posting, to me, seemed so abrupt that I kept scanning the archives to make sure I hadn't missed something. It was only after she posted this news that Amy began to dive more deeply into her emotions surrounding adoption and the simultaneous joy and pain she was carrying with her. Amy wrote about her feelings of pain and loss over expanding her family through adoption and not another pregnancy. While she was confident in her decision, for her health and their family's well-being, she was also grieving. She listed the things that she would miss out on (giving birth, feeling the baby move inside of her) but also the things that she would gain (finding out the gender before birth, having a new baby placed into her arms, looking into his or her eyes for the first time). She explained the dissonance between logic and emotion in this situation, writing, "This is not to say though that I am questioning adoption—not at all. I think adoption and dealing with never having another birth by choice are two different things, and I am working on each one."[7]

She is honest in admitting, "It still hurts."[8]

In May 2011, Amy wrote about a topic that hits extremely close to home for me. In a post titled "More Babies," she talks about the sadness she feels when she sees other women who are pregnant who'd had babies at the same time that she'd had her daughter.[9] Once again, she employs dialectical thinking (and I have to wonder whether she even knows she's doing it; I commend her for her insight and bravery), saying that she knows that there's no way she could handle another baby, especially so soon after her healing process, but, at the same time, she wishes it could be her. She touches on something I hadn't thought of previously—a hidden challenge of adoption. In summary, Amy explains that when you choose adoption, people make assumptions and sometimes ask for the story. Most people assume that there's a fertility or medical problem, so in sharing the true reason behind her choice to adopt, she would have to reveal her mental illness, perhaps at times when she was unprepared to. Her medical history is really no one's business, but as I know well, that doesn't stop people from asking.

So it's quite generous that Amy chose to share her story widely, first in her blog and later in that 2012 *Postpartum Progress* post. In it she wrote of her ongoing struggle and increasing ability to find acceptance:

> I still battle anxiety and depression that was brought on by the PPD, but it is no longer PPD. We have chosen to not get pregnant again because of the severity of my postpartum depression, so we are on the waiting list of adopting our next baby! That in itself was the hardest decision to make—choosing not to become pregnant again and feeling like I was broken, no good, choosing second best and a failure.
>
> I'd like to assure women that everyone will have a different journey and every woman will have different symptoms. I'd like to encourage women that they are not damaged or different, that they are not failures as moms or wives. Guilt can be a very damaging aspect of PPD; I am proof of that.[10]

A few months after the *Postpartum Progress* article was published, Amy took a hiatus from her own blog, and on August 4, 2013, she returned, writing, "It's been a long time—so much has happened," with "so much" including the birth and adoption of her new son, Lucas.[11] These new posts were filled with happiness and gratitude and so much love that it nearly jumped off the screen. She wrote proudly about her new son, who was then just a month shy of turning one year old (she first met him when he was just three days old, in September 2012). "Lucas has brought the most joy, the most amazing joy, to my life," she wrote. "He has been like a healer to my soul, when it was at the deepest pit of pain and [loneliness]."[12]

In the subsequent years, she acknowledged adoption as the greatest gift and as a source of endless fulfillment for her family.

In February 2018, Amy shared an emotional story that, fortunately, had a very happy ending. In a post called "A Year Ago Our World Turned Upside Down," Amy wrote that in 2017 she and her husband had endured two failed adoption matches: in each case, they had been told that they would be adopting a baby girl, and both times the birth parents changed their minds, deciding to keep the babies. After all of Amy's pain, and thinking that adoption would be her salve, she was subjected to even more heartache. But then, on what turned out to be an almost magical day, their old adoption caseworker called her cell phone unexpectedly, explaining that a baby boy was being born, literally at that moment, and asking whether Amy and her husband would like to adopt him. And so it was that one year later Amy could share with her readers the added joy that their new son, Josiah, was bringing to their world.[13]

Amy writes with great honesty, explaining the trials and tribulations that are part of the adoption process, for both the parents and all of the children involved. They had to work hard as a family to tend to each other's emotional needs. But in the end, Amy expanded her family, growing from one child to three, one by way of biology, two by way of adoption, and all with tremendous love.

There are so many wonderful reasons why adoption has felt right for our family, and then there are reasons that, to me, feel more selfish—harder to admit. We had always assumed that were we to adopt a child, as opposed to my carrying our biological child, I would not be at risk for medical or mental complications. I would not have prenatal anxiety or depression, nor would I be at risk for further postpartum depression or distress. I would not have to have a third cesarean section, so there would be no risk of uterine rupture or any of the other scary things that can happen when a uterus has a profile like mine.

Interestingly, despite our assumptions, studies and journal articles report cases of adoptive parents suffering from "postpartum depression." Though I am not a clinician, I am not sure that these articles have correctly labeled the affliction; I wonder whether what these families are suffering would be more appropriately termed "depression." The symptoms of postpartum depression and general depression are so similar, except that the mood changes in PPD are found in women who have just birthed a child and are therefore facing rapid and robust hormonal fluctuations. While I understand the reasoning behind calling depression after adoption "postpartum depression," I also find it misleading. To me, it would be like my saying that any depression I suffer today is postpartum depression today; technically I am postpregnancy (albeit five years postpregnancy).

Nonetheless, one study out of Purdue University addressing "parental depression in the postadoption time periods" claims that "parents express unfulfilled and unrealistic expectations in the domains of self, child, family or friends, and society or others."[14]

Despite some of my initial reservations with the article, I appreciate the author's insistence that parents seek support and help. "We need to empower parents," Karen Foli writes, "to share their feelings with adoption-smart professionals, online or face-to-face support groups, trusted significant others, and friends. Parents should realize they are not being disloyal to their children or families to feel the way they do. Healthcare providers . . . can be instrumental in detecting issues related to depression or the mental well-being of the parents. Being more open about such concerns can lead to a healthier, happier family. By helping themselves, they are helping their children."[15]

Several years later, in 2012, Foli, an adoptive mother herself, found that postadoption depression syndrome—or PADS, as it is known—is not uncommon, "although it's not as well documented as postpartum depression." In fact, Foli found that "between 18 and 26 percent of adoptive mothers (depending on the screening scale) reported depressive symptoms within the first year of bringing home a new baby or child."[16]

Another study clarifies the similarities and dissimilarities between postpartum depression and postadoption depression. "Because increased stress is linked to depression during the postpartum period," the researchers write, "women who adopt children may be also at risk for developing depression. Postpartum and adoptive women may experience similar life changes; however, the stressors associated with having a biological child may be different from stressors associated with adopting a child."[17]

In learning this information, my head swam and my heart sank. Please don't get me wrong: never have I ever had the notion that adoption would be easy. I knew that adoption would have a significant psychological impact on each one of our family members, including a prospective adopted child—our child. I was naive, however, in thinking that adoption would spare me from the severe mental-health struggles I'd suffered after Beau's birth. While I would not have the raging hormones to contend with, I would have other, new anxieties, concerns, pressures, and woes. I would feel alienated and confused in entirely new ways.

Armed with all of this new information, I came to Kenny to, once again, discuss our options. I told him about postadoption depression and how, despite our hopes, adoption would not, in fact, mitigate my risk for future mental-health issues related to having another baby. His reply was insightful and clear.

"Having a baby is stressful. There's the lack of sleep, the change in your daily schedule, the immense responsibility, and an infinite number of other things that, when you put them together, of course can lead to depression. I'm not a professional, but this makes sense to me." He allayed some of my new fears by validating them and also understanding them. Like all things, once they were spoken, they became less powerful.

One of the most important things to me throughout this entire should-we-expand-our-family journey has been remaining a united front with Kenny. On an obvious level, when it comes to making a significant, life-changing decision—and one that will impact not only our family but also our marriage—it is incredibly important to me that we feel like a team. Our marriage is stronger now than ever, but it took a lot of hard, scary work to get to this place. My postpartum depression took a toll on us as a couple, and I would never want to consciously set up any additional roadblocks for us.

But on a deeper level, unity in this decision is something that I don't just want but, rather, need. When Kenny changed his mind about wanting another child, it not only made me feel grateful to him as a husband and father but also made me feel loved. Perhaps this is childish or selfish or immature, but it further cements us together.

It's why the six purple hearts served to symbolize so much for me.

I want to be clear in saying that this would not be, in any way, a "reconciliation baby" or "redo baby." We are solid and have nothing to redo. And in terms of commitment, while Kenny and I are legally bound, we also already have a daughter, a son, a house, several pets, and a large extended family that keep us connected. It's safe to say that, new baby or not, we're both in this.

The same way that I wanted Beau to want another baby, I have always wanted Kenny to want another baby even more. If we do decide to expand our family, I need Kenny to commit to keep pulling on the rope, even when I get tired. If I lose my way, I need for him to redirect me. He knows where I want to go, and I need to trust that he'll get me there, even when the trek feels arduous and frightening.

Adoption is an incredibly special way to expand a family after postpartum depression. Though it's costly and emotionally taxing and can come with its own set of mental-health issues, it can be supremely beneficial for so many of the people involved in the process. The idea that I could provide a child with a good home is staggering to me in its power. Truthfully, it would be an honor. Though there are things that feel big or scary or overwhelming about adoption, I have to remind myself that there were things that felt big or scary or overwhelming when I first got pregnant, as it was so new. Frankly, if I were to get pregnant again, there would be so many things that would feel big and scary and overwhelming. Would a child feel strange about being adopted when his siblings were not?

Who's to say? There's no guarantee that a biological child would feel a greater or lesser sense of belonging in our family.

Like most things, adoption would be a leap of faith. But with an upside potentially so miraculous, it seems like one to which we could be *open*.

6

❖ ❖

Open for Occupancy:
Surrogacy After Postpartum
Depression

Belle and I, having donned our "cozy clothes," cuddled up in my bed on an unseasonably warm Friday night.

"I want to read something to you," I told her. "Please be honest; I promise you won't hurt my feelings," I instructed, using my most gentle, loving voice.

I had just written the rough manuscript for a children's book, aimed to normalize feelings for young kids, and I needed my best test subject.

She snuggled up with me as I read the story to her, in long, picture-book form, using deliberate repetition and vivid metaphors.

I read her the story of a mother and daughter who, through the years, lived an enchanted life together. They caught snowflakes on their tongues, rubbed their cold, red noses together, jumped in big puddles during rainstorms, collected sea glass at the ocean's edge, climbed on swing sets to play as pirates, and then, every night, cuddled up together for a bedtime story.

The message of the story was that no person, no adult and no child, would be happy all the time. And that that is okay.

That we all have feelings, and some of them are happy, and some of them are sad, and some feelings are strong and powerful and don't even have names.

When I finished reading the story, Belle had tears pooled in her eyes, which started to roll down her cheek; she looked almost like a cartoon character. She has my big, ever-expressive eyes, and in them I can see, and in them I can feel.

"I love it, Mommy," she said, blinking back the tears.

"How did it make you feel?" I asked, pulling her body into mine and positioning her into the nook I had created between the crook of my arm and my chest.

"I think I feel one of those feelings that doesn't have a name," she started, quietly. She is so wise. "It didn't make me sad, so don't worry that I am crying sad, but it also just feels like my heart is being tugged."

She slays me.

"Maybe," I offered, "what you are feeling is moved?"

She nodded, wordlessly, and continued to burrow her head into the special spot in my body that is only hers.

Belle is a feeler—an empath. She and I go through life with big emotions, and it has made life more vibrant and more colorful and more delicious and more beautiful, and at the same time it can also make life harder. Fully embracing one's emotions is difficult for adults to master, let alone an eight-year-old, but my eight-year-old is an old soul.

She does not just hear music; rather, she feels music. I understand this because I do the same.

We do this thing, together, where we listen to a song, and while we listen we hold hands. When one of us feels a part of the music that makes our heart swell or makes our stomach do flip-flops, we squeeze the other's hand (as to not interrupt the song by speaking). For someone who does not feel music in the way we do, this exercise would not make sense and, perhaps, seem silly. For anyone who does feel music in the way we do, you are welcome.

Belle and I are not scared of vulnerability. Yes, vulnerability may make the hurty things hurt, but it makes the beautiful things feel electrifying.

With her head on my chest, Belle wrapped her arms around me, her small hand lingering on my stomach.

She poked at it and said, "Squishy!"—a sobering reminder that while she is an old soul, she is also still a child and often lacks a filter.

She's right, though, in that my stomach is squishy. To be more accurate, it is the skin on my stomach area, so stretched during my pregnancies, that now hangs loosely, while also being adorned with stretch marks for good measure.

I remind her of this when she expresses her confusion about this part of my body that hardly anyone is allowed to see.

"Mommy, if you have another baby, I have an idea for a gender reveal."

Her abrupt pivot, at a time when we were both already feeling so unzipped, hit me so hard that I felt as if I had experienced whiplash.

The idea of a third child had been floating in the air for months ever since Kenny and I had begun dancing around it—and let our children in on it.

Because I had just made a point of explaining to Belle why it's so important to normalize all feelings, I didn't think it would be right to shut this conversation down, but I knew that I was wading into treacherous (moat-like) water.

Having been unzipped by the story I had written and shared with her, and having held her in my arms, and given that she and I had both been so moved, I would feel everything more acutely. And the baby topic always feels big to me. I did not want to burden her with my feelings, nor did I think it was appropriate to stifle them, for me or for her, so I let her speak and held back my own tears from behind my own cartoon-character-like eyes.

She went on to tell me her latest ideas for a gender reveal—which, really, were like four different gender-reveal activities in one, involving things like colored cupcakes into which guests would bite, balloons that would be released from a box and/or filled with confetti before being pricked with a pin, and slime that would be dumped onto my head.

On she went, chatting about her preferences, in nuanced, complicated ways.

"I think I would be happiest if I saw pink icing or pink balloons, because I really like pink, but I actually want a baby brother, so I would want the balloons to be blue; I just don't like blue as much. Could we do different colors? Like rose gold and frozen gold? That way I can be excited about the color *and* I can also be excited about it being a boy or a girl? I really don't care either way, except if I *had* to choose, I would want another little brother, because if I picture myself walking down the aisle with Beau at someone's wedding, I imagine him as the ring bearer, and I see myself as the flower girl, and I don't see another girl as a flower girl with me, but I can imagine a little baby boy with Beau."

Another similarity between us is that Belle's mind, like mine, moves at warp speed. Fortunately, as exhausting as it can be, I speak Belle and followed her exact train of thought.

And, as predicted, it began to cause me pain.

My glassy eyes started to fill up, more and more, at the image of a family photo in which we had our two children and another little baby, dressed in a tiny suit and pair of dress shoes. My heart began to ache. I could see the picture so vividly, but, once again, I got so stuck when I thought of the logistics around it.

"How are we having this baby?"

and

"Would it really be this happy for us?"

and

"Whose wedding is this, anyway?"

At first, I didn't want her to see me crying.

But as the tears continued to fall, I looked down at my daughter. My brown-eyed girl—sensitive and sweet and determined girl. My Belle.

I looked at her bow-like lips, and my heart fell into my stomach, in a way that was both good and hard at the same time.

"Mommy?" Belle came back to reality. "Are you sad? Did I make you sad?"

"It's okay," I told her, whispering the words as I swallowed my tears. "No, Lovey, you did not make me sad. You are amazing."

"Are you just feeling moved like the mommy in the story?"

I nodded my head, and she stretched her neck, her face now pressed against my own. She rubbed her little nose against mine, just like the characters in the story, who, in all honesty, are just like us, and she squeezed me.

"It's okay, Mommy. It's okay to feel! We all have feelings!"

She got me there.

In that moment, I thought of a different picture in my mind. It was of Belle and Beau meeting their new little sibling. They were a little older, and the baby's head was covered in a hospital hat, which was always my favorite of all of the hats, and its body was wrapped in a hospital swaddling blanket.

"It's okay, little baby. Don't cry!" I heard her voice, using the same words she used when she first met her brother, so many lifetimes ago—the same words she had just said to me, in bed, on a quiet Friday night.

A familiar feeling of warmth spread from my chest and into my stomach. It was an uncomfortable feeling, like a longing. I think I was simultaneously nostalgic and wistful for the days that had passed and yearning for the days that had yet to come—but that, I realized, might never come.

I knew that Belle's and my conversation could send us shooting down a rabbit hole, and, as the adult, I had to reroute us and to put us back on steady ground. As much as I wanted to go into Belle's world with her and to dream up gender-reveal parties and ask her about baby names and continue to imagine a life in which the decisions had been made and a baby was in my arms, it was not the time. It would not be fair to her.

"Mommy," I could hear. I recognized the voice as I tried to shake it from my head.

It was the baby, from far away, by the castle, across the moat.

I had to drown it out if I wanted to salvage my evening with Belle, and so I scooped my little girl up in my arms, my last tears wiped away from my cheeks.

"Do you want to have a hot cocoa date?" I asked her with a smile that was only partially fake.

"Yes!" she squealed.

As we walked out of the room and down the stairs, the baby's voice got further and further away.

"Don't worry," I said to the baby voice in my mind. "I am not leaving you. I am working on this. Be patient. Mommy is here."

And I turned on the stove to boil water for our cocoa.

In the years following Beau's birth, once my postpartum depression had stabilized, I spent a lot of time trying to process and grieve the loss of my ability to have more children.

As I wrote in my first book,

> Sometimes I have dreams that the doctor was wrong, that I can, actually, decide to "try" again. I can wait, with a quickened heartbeat, for two lines to appear on a stick. I can see a little teddy bear–shaped person flickering on an ultrasound. I can find out if the baby is a boy or a girl. I can feel kicks and feel nauseated and feel the baby being pulled from inside of me as I hear the doctor say, "I see a hand! I see a foot!"
>
> Sometimes I feel angry, at my body and at my brain chemistry and at my doctors. I am angry that this happened to me.
>
> Other times I ask my husband if, in six years, assuming we have loads of money, we could hire a surrogate to carry a third baby for us. Bargaining.
>
> And then there's the depression. The part of me that is making my eyes sting now as I type these words.
>
> I am waiting for the acceptance.[1]

The notion of a surrogate is one that I have explored in my consciousness for the past several years and has been, in many ways, the most appealing option for me. It is, however, not without its risks, financial burdens, and the need for a level of trust that I am not sure I can have in any other human. Having another woman carry our child, in my mind, solves so many of our problems, answers so many questions, and gives us an option that feels both safe for me and comfortable for the future child. We could expand our family without putting my body or brain at risk. Having a baby that grows in someone else's womb would eliminate the need for me to undergo another C-section, which is major abdominal surgery and something that still scares me very much. A surrogate would also eliminate the risk of my developing prenatal or postpartum depression, which, as we know, can be life threatening and is something that still scares my loved ones very much.

I have always had some rudimentary knowledge of what *surrogacy* means. I always thought that by using a surrogate we would have to used assisted reproductive technology (ART) and that Kenny and I would create an embryo, with his sperm and my egg, just like we had done with our IVF process with Dr. G, and that the doctors would then implant that embryo into another woman's uterus. If the implantation were successful, this woman would be the one to carry and deliver the baby, and it would, from start to finish, be ours. What I have learned, in my extensive conversations with those who have used surrogates and gestational carriers, and those who have served as surrogates and gestational carriers, is that there is a major difference between a *surrogate* and a *gestational carrier* despite the fact that the terms are often thrown around interchangeably.

In the case of a surrogate, a woman donates her own egg, which is then fertilized by a man's sperm, and then she subsequently carries the child. She is genetically, biologically tied to the baby she carries but is not the intended parent. In many cases, this is referred to as *traditional surrogacy*, and the woman would be called a *traditional surrogate*.

By contrast, a gestational carrier is a woman who is implanted with an embryo using IVF, created from the egg from another woman and the sperm from a man, and she carries and delivers the baby without any genetic or biological link to the child whatsoever. This is even more nuanced, as in the case of a gestational carrier there are many scenarios that account for the genetics of the future child. When using a gestational-surrogacy approach, the embryo with which she is implanted could be one that is 100 percent biologically related to the intended parents. The embryo could also be created from a donor sperm and donor egg, just not that from the carrier, so that it is not genetically linked to either the carrier or the intended parents. And in some cases the embryo has been created using the intended mother's egg combined with donor sperm, or the intended father's sperm and a donor egg. And that is the least complicated part!

I remember times when, during my active postpartum depression, both my best friend and my sister offered their wombs to me. My best friend was not yet a mother and said that as long as pregnancy went well for her, she would carry a baby for me. She is a very loving, giving friend. My sister, who does not yet have children of her own, has also told me that I could rent space in her uterus for nine months. She is a very loving, giving sister. In these cases, my best friend or sister would serve as my gestational carrier. I still bring this up with them today, and I think they think I am joking, and I don't think they realize that I'm not.

In trying to find information on the practice of surrogacy for family expansion after postpartum depression, I had to wade through a sea of articles on postpartum depression in the gestational carrier. I found one Internet article on a site called *Babygaga*, titled "15 Reasons to Opt for a Surrogate." Reason number eleven is "Risk of postpartum depression," and the article goes on to explain, "The fear and anxiety of that can keep families from expanding the way they want to. If a family is struggling with the reality of PPD but still have the desire to have more children, then they should consider gestational or traditional surrogacy." While I was relieved to see this option represented in mainstream media, I cannot ignore the fact that reason number fourteen on said list is "Fear the baby will be ugly," with a horrifyingly offensive accompanying picture of a baby photoshopped to look like it has the face of a dog.[2]

Other articles on the topic were equally offensive, if not more so.

In a roundabout way to find more data on the subject, I researched "reasons why people choose surrogacy" and, like the previous articles mentioned, was met with many lists. Often these lists did not mention any mental-health issues, let alone postpartum depression.

In fact, in two separate articles published by the incredibly popular online American women's magazine *Bustle*, the reasons why a woman might choose a surrogate were solely limited to medical conditions, including infertility, previous miscarriages, and a prior hysterectomy.[3] Considering that the site has nearly five million social media followers and, according to the ever-reliable bastion of truth Wikipedia, gets more than ten million unique visitors per month, I find this omission insensitive.

Where does a woman turn when she is considering a surrogate after having postpartum depression? In circles, evidently.

While the idea of traditional surrogacy and gestational surrogacy have always seemed appealing to me, in practice, as many things are, it is much more complex. According to WebMD, among the reasons people consider surrogacy are "conditions that make pregnancy impossible or risky" for the mother.[4]

The first surrogacy using ART, in which a surrogate mother was implanted with, carried, and gave birth to a baby (for compensation) with whom she had no biological relation, occurred with a pregnancy in 1985 and subsequent birth in 1986.[5]

US laws around both surrogacy and gestational carriers are complicated and mercurial and vary greatly between states (on a spectrum ranging from "surrogacy friendly" to states that ban the practice outright). Intuitively, surrogacy is more legally complex than gestational carrying, as the woman who carries the baby is also biologically related to the child, which brings up a myriad of emotional and legal issues for all parties involved. My reaction to this situation is that surrogacy must be really, really hard.

I can imagine it being hard for a surrogate mother who chooses to get pregnant with, carry, and deliver a baby to whom she is genetically related and then not serve as its parent. The concoction made of hormones and biological factors in that situation seems like a recipe for difficulty—not insurmountable and not universally complicated, but potentially so. I can also see surrogacy being difficult for the baby's own intended parents; if the child is biologically related to the woman who carried the baby and went through the experience of giving birth, I can imagine a range of complex emotions being felt by all.

Because of the genetic link with all surrogacy situations, prospective parents need to have a signed *birth order*, which is the legal document that ascribes parentage to a baby. There are prebirth order agreements, which allow parents to assume parental rights starting in the fourth month of pregnancy and are fully executed by the seventh month of pregnancy.

Postbirth order agreements, required by some states, are signed in court in the days immediately following the baby's birth. Being a Pennsylvania resident, I feel lucky to be in a state that uses prebirth order agreements,[6] but once I told Kenny about this part of surrogacy, one of the many legal aspects about which we were unaware, his response was an eloquent and explicable "Whoa."

It appears that we are not alone in our reaction to the complexities of traditional surrogacy, as, according to WebMD, "gestational surrogacy has become more common than a traditional surrogate." It reports that approximately 750 babies are born in the United States each year by way of gestational surrogacy.[7]

The data surrounding traditional surrogacy, however, are much harder to unveil. According to the Council for Responsible Genetics, a "nonprofit, nongovernmental organization" that "represents the public interest and fosters public debate about the social, ethical, and environmental implications of genetic technologies," statistics about traditional surrogacy have not yet been reliably reported to the public.[8] Their estimate was that between 2004 and 2008, in the United States an average of nine children were born in every state, each year, by way of surrogacy, though this statistic is not broken down between traditional surrogacy and gestational surrogacy. The data do, however, show the rising popularity in surrogate births in the past decade.

Before exploring personal, specific options, I decided that it would behoove me to become more knowledgeable about the surrogacy process in general in Pennsylvania so that I could be as informed as I have been with every other step of my journey. Though surrogacy seemed prohibitively expensive, I considered it a valid, valuable choice and wanted to understand it as thoroughly as possible.[9]

The first thing that I discovered is that there is far more information available for prospective surrogate mothers and gestational carriers than there is for prospective intended parents. I encountered countless websites that appeared to be of "general interest" but actually contained heaps of information for women considering this life choice; they were almost always connected to a law firm.

These websites lay out the general terms that should be included in a surrogacy agreement, like terms for parental rights, custody, location of delivery, future contact between the parties' health-insurance companies, insurance obligations, medical decisions during pregnancy (who will make them and how), payment of medical bills, liability for medical complications (if any), financial considerations in supporting the gestational carrier (compensation, expenses, lost wages, legal fees, childcare, maternity clothing, insurance, etc.), the provision of medical history and personal information, continued contact between the gestational carrier and intended parents (including during medical office visits and the baby's delivery), and informed consent.

In Pennsylvania, strict laws dictate who can be a gestational carrier. Lisa Marie Vari, a family law and divorce attorney in Pittsburgh, explains:

A Pennsylvania woman who is considering acting as a gestational surrogate should have (or lack as the case may be) the following characteristics:

1. The gestational surrogate (sometimes referred to as a carrier) should be between twenty-one and forty-five years of age;
2. The gestational carrier [would] have at least one full term and uncomplicated pregnancy;
3. The surrogate should have no more than five previous births;
4. The gestational surrogate should have no more than three previous cesarean section births;
5. The gestational carrier should not have a history of [postpartum] depression;
6. The surrogate should be raising her children in her home and not have had any allegations of child abuse or child protective services oversight of her parental relationship with her children;
7. The surrogate mother should have a stable family environment and adequate emotional support system to help her through the surrogacy process;
8. The surrogate carrier should have a healthy body mass index of thirty or less and have healthy eating habits;
9. The gestational surrogate should not smoke, use illicit drugs, or consume alcohol on a regular basis;
10. The surrogate mother should not be receiving public assistance benefits as the payment arrangements under a surrogacy contract may disqualify the surrogate from continued benefits including cash assistance or housing benefits;
11. Ideally, the carrier should have private medical insurance coverage [that] does not exclude medical costs associated with surrogacy. If a medical exclusion in a private health insurance policy exists, a surrogacy insurance contract may be available or the intended parents must privately pay all costs associated with the IVF or other process, prenatal, and delivery costs. Public assistance benefits will generally not provide coverage under surrogacy arrangements;
12. The gestational carrier should have [adequate] transportation to and from medical screenings and appointments and any mental health evaluations or joint counseling sessions;
13. The surrogate should be free from any antidepressants or antianxiety medications for at least twelve months prior to the start of the surrogacy process;
14. The gestational surrogate should not have a criminal history of any [misdemeanor] or felony charges or convictions;
15. The carrier should have at least twelve months lapse since any piercings or tattoos;

16. The gestational carrier should not have any sexually transmitted diseases;
17. The gestational surrogate should not have unresolved or untreated major depression, [bipolar] disorder, psychosis, significant anxiety disorder, or personality disorder; and
18. The surrogate should not have unresolved or untreated [addiction], child abuse [issues], sexual or physical abuse [issues], depression, or eating [disorders].

What will disqualify a woman from acting as a gestational surrogate in Pennsylvania? . . .

Standard protocols when considering the use of a gestational carrier in Pennsylvania include medical screening and testing of a potential surrogate as well as social, behavioral, and psychological screening and testing.[10]

With everything I learned about surrogacy, I had several simultaneous, visceral reactions. First, I was completely overwhelmed by the layers (and legality) involved with the surrogacy process. Second, I was completely overcome with admiration for those who go through it.

Third, and perhaps most relevantly, I was absolutely stunned to read all of the legal requirements that would disqualify *me* as a surrogate mother or gestational carrier. I have a history of postpartum depression. While my BMI is under thirty, it is not within the healthy range; rather, it is below it. Not only would I not be free of any antidepressants or antianxiety medications for twelve months prior to pregnancy, but I would be actively, deliberately, *thoughtfully* staying on my antidepressant during a future pregnancy. If I would not qualify to carry someone else's child, am I not qualified to carry my own?

This realization fell onto me like an itchy blanket slung over my shoulders. Except, unlike those scratchy, woolen throws, I could not get it off.

What does it mean to be a mother? This is a question I have asked myself, on repeat, over the years. But like many questions that have an abundance of answers, here there are even more questions.

Not only did my research on surrogacy taint my notion of biological motherhood, but it also got me thinking about a potential gestational carrier and the risks to her mental health. What happens to the surrogate mothers who carry these babies, deliver them, and then, presumably, vanish into the night? What about the gestational carriers' mental health? If I were to use a gestational carrier in order to bring another child into our family (a phrase that makes me cringe, in that the term "use" is so often *used* in this situation, but it feels, at best, so utilitarian and, at worst, so demoralizing) and, in doing so, send her flying down the avalanche that is postpartum depression, how could I ever forgive myself?

The questions never cease.

In scouring the Internet, social media channels, and my own personal networks, I had an extremely difficult time finding any information on mothers who have chosen to pursue surrogacy, either traditional surrogacy or with a gestational carrier, after postpartum depression. Like many things, surrogacy is, sadly, still stigmatized in this country. The notion of mental-health issues coupled with surrogacy is a double whammy, and so it has been swept under the proverbial nursery rug, and these stories seem to have been written in private diaries as opposed to major news outlets or in the blogosphere.

I did come across one story that resonated deeply with me, from an August 2012 message board on *The Bump*, a very popular online website about pregnancy and babies (affiliated with the perpetually popular wedding-planning website, *The Knot*). I found the story of a woman who calls herself "MrsBraun," though I do not know whether this is her real name. She writes a post under the subheading of "Adoption," titled "Postpartum Depression Leads to Finding a Surrogate—Here's My Story." Her story is so similar to mine in some ways, as we both had our first child, daughters, in 2010, and so different in others. After her daughter's birth, she writes, she "suffered *severe* postpartum depression" and "was hospitalized for over six months." During her struggle, MrsBraun received electroconvulsive therapy (ECT) for depression and even had her daughter taken from her temporarily because she "couldn't cope with her in the house." She continues, "I was told never to have children again because I could risk my life or the life of the newborn. At the time I thought, 'Thank goodness' because *why* would I *ever* want to go through this again?! The thought of it made me [nauseated]."[11]

MrsBraun explains that now, two years later, the thought of never having any more children breaks her heart; she dreams about it all the time and would love to see her daughter as an older sibling. After finding adoption a prohibitively expensive option, she and her husband "fell in love with the idea" of traditional surrogacy. Her husband's sperm would artificially inseminate the woman's egg, and the woman would carry and deliver the baby for MrsBraun and her husband. And so MrsBraun was turning to the message board to ask for advice. She had questions about attachment—or the lack thereof. She wondered whether she would feel resentful, either toward her husband or, potentially, toward a new child. She asked for help figuring out how to prepare for this journey.[12]

She received nine responses to her query, ranging from simple "I support you!"–type messages to real answers, using data and personal experiences. It was through the replies, and MrsBraun's answers to said replies, that I learned that, although she would have elected to do a gestational surrogacy, where another woman would carry a baby that was biologically her own, it was, like adoption, exceedingly costly.[13]

One commenter, known as "Kaitylin," a member of the *The Bump* since 2008, wrote in response to MrsBraun's post, sharing her own story of severe postpartum anxiety and its impact on her ability to have future children of her own. Kaitylin wrote that she kept her severe prenatal and postpartum anxiety from her loved ones, even paying out of pocket for fifteen secret prenatal ultrasounds to check on the health of her growing baby. And yet, like MrsBraun, and myself, Kaitylin was having a terribly difficult time letting go of the idea of future family expansion. As she explains, "I am completely terrified of the idea of going back to that place and having the anxiety again[.] I don't know yet if we will . . . I'm hoping I'll be able to as all my doctors feel confident the anxiety is resolved (I am off all medication). I'm not sure if maybe in five to seven years we will try again, but I will definitely be on the lookout for issues and will address any anxiety much sooner . . . I want to wait until [my darling daughter] is old enough that I won't have the stress of a toddler and newborn."[14]

The secret sisterhood of the severe sufferers.

For what it's worth, Kaitylin has posted on *The Bump* more than 1.6 thousand times over the years but has yet to post about a subsequent pregnancy, surrogacy, or adoption situation in the seven years since her exchange with MrsBraun.

MrsBraun, however, did. Later that month, MrsBraun posted a query on the site—"Crazy Question—Anyone Here Use a Surrogate??"—sharing that she and her husband were doing their first cycle of artificial insemination, and she was looking to find some camaraderie. In her post, she opens up, completely candidly, by announcing that they are using a traditional surrogate (as she had mentioned previously) and refers to the surrogate as the biological mom of the baby. Despite her initial reservations, she is "super duper excited!" but also feels "weird" because it's like she's the one going through all the pregnancy testing, worrying about the positive or negative results. "It's an odd feeling, but it's something that has to be done." She then asks whether anyone on the site has had any experience with a surrogate or, conversely, whether anyone is curious about the process and wants to ask her for advice.[15]

Despite her offer to share, among the seven replies she received to her post, she received two questions posed to her by two different women, and she never responded. The first question was from a mother who had also longed to be a surrogate herself, asking MrsBraun whether she picked her own surrogate or if the surrogate had chosen her. The second question asked why MrsBraun had chosen to go the "surrogate route" and how she chose the surrogate they would be using.[16]

MrsBraun's final query on *The Bump* was—in my eyes—unexpected, to put it delicately. It was posted at the end of the same month during which she had first asked about surrogacy as an option, and it is not clear whether the pregnancy has even been achieved at the time of said posting. Her post, now under the "Parenting" umbrella of the message boards, is titled "Random—Would You Name Your Child After Your Surrogate??"[17]

In (rather) stark contrast with her initial question, filled with worries about resentment and connection, she is now asking the community whether she should use the surrogate's name (which she reveals is Dawn) as the middle name for their future child, if said child is a female. According to MrsBraun, they have a "great relationship" with Dawn and plan to continue to have her in their lives, even after the birth of their child. She ponders whether using Dawn as the child's middle name is potentially too personal, or perhaps confusing, as her plan is to tell the child, when the child is deemed old enough, "that Dawn is a close friend that carried" him or her but that Dawn is actually also the biological mother, though she leaves room for them to change their minds when the time comes.[18]

In her post, MrsBraun also expresses concern that *Dawn* rhymes with *Braun*—or, as she puts it, the names are "a little too matchy-matchy," and so would it be okay to give this child two middle names? To this question she received fourteen replies, the most out of any of her posts, and they were almost all exclusively negative in one way or another. Some specifically addressed the idea of naming the baby after the surrogate, and others addressed using a surrogate at all, expressing judgment and telling MrsBraun that she would only be the child's adopted mother, questioning her as to why she would not use her own eggs. Interestingly, however, two of the comments were about surrogacy, one from a potential intended parent and the other from a potential surrogate carrier.[19]

A woman going by the name of "ABColeslaw" shared that her family was trying to grow by way of a gestational surrogate and that she was hopeful that their dreams would be realized in the future. ABColeslaw writes that with a gestational surrogate the baby will be biologically created by herself and her husband. "However, absolutely, I would totally consider using our surrogate's name. I would never stop loving the woman who would give my family that gift. And I would love having my daughter carry that name." I could relate to her sentiment profoundly, as I cannot think of many gifts as generous as the gift of a womb for a future child. Though ABColeslaw clarifies things with the caveat ". . . provided I liked the name."[20]

Throughout this process, I had the privilege of connecting with several amazing women who have served or currently are serving as both surrogates and gestational carriers. As I marveled at their social media pages, all filled with positivity and generosity, I was overcome with gratitude that people like this—people with so much love in their hearts—exist. The women I met care deeply for the babies they carry and feel the weight of the responsibility, knowing how important their role is in building families for those who otherwise could not.

The first woman with whom I became virtually acquainted is named Christine. She is a wife, mother, and surrogate gestational carrier, and I first learned about her story on Instagram. It should be noted that social media outlets are now forums on which people can connect, personally, to aid in the family-expansion pursuit, so my finding her on Instagram is not at all unusual; intended parents can find their surrogates, birth mothers can look at the profiles of potential adoptive parents, and an author can find research subjects for her book on family expansion after postpartum depression, all online.

Christine has been chronicling her journey as a surrogate gestational carrier and uses her page *Stork Stories* as a "diary" where she posts photos, extensive captions, detailed videos, and an incredible amount of heart, which all jumps off the screen. She refers to herself as a "stork" because she, in essence, delivers babies, all created and carried and cared for, to their forever families—just like the mythical birds in the age-old stories who drop sweet, little bundles on people's doorsteps. I was first drawn to Christine when I saw a photo she'd posted of a young woman with a broad smile holding a tiny baby next to a letter board that read "Womb Empty/ Heart Full." I would learn that Christine, the mother of two biological children of her own, decided to become a surrogate carrier to help other families to expand. Though the story of the stork is, of course, a fictional tale, filled with magic and enchantment, it does mimic much of what Christine is able to do for intended parents; it's just a little less fairy-tale-y or feathery.[21]

I sent Christine a direct message on Instagram, and she responded promptly and kindly. I thanked her for what she does to help others and asked whether she would be willing to speak to me, both as a mother looking to potentially expand my family and as an author, exploring this option for a book.

"Sure! I'm always up for helping others if I can," she replied.

As soon as we connected, I praised Christine for her positive attitude and bountiful generosity.

"You are too kind," she said, humbly. "To be honest, I'm not completely selfless in this. There is great reward in helping a family grow. My family wasn't too excited about me doing this again, but I really pushed to be a part of something greater than us. Of course they are extremely supportive, *but* I immediately felt I wasn't done after the first surrogacy journey."

I was so struck by the last part of her message.

Christine, who had carried and delivered two children of her own, and then carried and delivered another baby for another couple, was, in many ways, in the exact same position that I am in: she feels, deeply and strongly, that she is not done with her journey, that her story is not complete.

Her explanation is so evocative. I know that my feeling of being incomplete is hard to comprehend for many, especially since I already have two children. Like I've said before, it's no different for me than it is for a woman or man who longs to have a first child; the differences and nuances are in the details. Christine and I have an unspoken kinship. She feels destined for future pregnancies; I feel destined for a future baby. We feel the same way. Just like I said, the differences are all in the details.

During her first surrogacy pregnancy, Christine called the baby inside of her womb her "belly buddy." I was amazed at how keenly skilled she appears at being such a loving carrier for this baby and, at the same time, being able to separate the fact that the baby is not, in fact, her own.

Six months after her first delivery as a surrogate gestational carrier Christine was medically cleared for another surrogate pregnancy. This involved removing adhesions from her uterus. As I suspected, being a surrogate gestational carrier is not a walk in the park and involves tremendous physical and emotional sacrifice (if not pain). But it's pretty extraordinary.

As I write, Christine is preparing for her second pregnancy as a ges-tational surrogate, and I'm watching the process, with both familiarity and wonder, as she shows the scores of medications, enormous pile of syringes, and videos of her receiving her initial rounds of injections. I have done this before, too. I know the sting of the long, subcutaneous and intra-muscular injections. But rather than complain, Christine posted an artistic photo, where in the background you can see the blurred-out image of nine pill bottles, countless needles, alcohol pads, and all of the other medical equipment. In the foreground, and perfectly in focus, she posted another letter board, on which she spelled out, "They say you can do anything you put your mind to so I became a *surrogate.*" To me, that says it all.

The next surrogate with whom I connected, also through Instagram, is named Michelle Griffin.[22] In the brief header on her Instagram page, Michelle describes herself as "Mother, Wife, Doula, Surrogate."

I was first taken with Michelle when I saw a post she created with the caption "Me vs other preggo ladies on [Instagram]" accompanying two photos, and she directs her followers to swipe in order to see both, with the use of a finger-pointing emoji. The photos, from afar, look identical: She's holding up a pink letter board with white letters over her face, while wearing a pale-pink sports bra and black bikini bottoms, her pregnant belly covered with yellow sticky notes. (It should be noted that letter boards have now become a motif in the story of surrogates on Instagram, but that's because letter boards, signs on which moveable and removable let-ters can be rearranged to spell messages, are currently one of the biggest trends on this particular social media platform.) In both of the photos, the letter board says, "*Can't wait to . . .*" and the notes are meant to complete the sentence. In the photo that Michelle uses to represent "other preggo people"—by which she means women who are carrying their own chil-dren with traditional pregnancies—the sticky notes, written in thick, black marker, read, "hold you," "kiss you," "meet you," "hug you," and "squeeze you." In the other photo, the notes read, "stop peeing every 5 [minutes]," "sleep properly," "have a cocktail," "be able to lift my kids again," and, most poignantly, right in the center of her pregnant belly, "see you with your parents," and she drew a heart under her words on that note. I found this touching, genuine, and surprisingly relatable. In all honesty, Michelle could have captioned this post something like "What you think you'll feel about pregnancy vs the truth about pregnancy," as her answers in the latter photo are refreshingly honest and, excepting the last note, could apply to many pregnant women who are both excited and uncomfortable.

Because Michelle is so relatable and open, when we connected I asked her a lot of questions about her experience with surrogacy, the process in general, and, most important to me, her feelings about it all.

In terms of logistics, Michelle explained, "We spent about a year going through the counseling sessions, [psychological] evaluations, lawyer consultations, and approval from the Reproductive Technology Council. It was a lengthy process, but it was very straight forward and so important to go through to make sure everyone was on the same page." Surrogacy seems daunting, and overwhelming, and so reading her honest account provided me with reassurance.

I asked Michelle how she was able to cope with the stressors, including the "fertility stuff," and her sincerity was evident in her reply. I asked her about this in particular as I had seen her post on Instagram, so transparently, the photos of the five pregnancy tests she took to confirm her surrogacy pregnancy, with a caption explaining that with her own children she solely took one pregnancy test, whereas with her current pregnancy she felt more responsible and was incredibly invested in the result. She shared, "I remember shaking and crying, being so overwhelmed that it finally worked!" They were, she says, "memories I'll cherish forever." She later explained to me, via e-mail, that despite having no fertility issues with her own children, it took her six months to do the embryo creation and then three transfers in order to become pregnant with the baby she's currently carrying. "This was tough because I had never had difficulty falling pregnant before so just assumed it would happen easily this time too. It was hard to let the whole team down twice, but luckily we fell pregnant on the third try, and it's been smooth sailing since."

I asked Michelle what piece of advice she would give to parents who are looking to expand their families after postpartum depression but cannot (or are hesitant to) by way of pregnancy and so instead are exploring surrogacy. Her answer was clear: she emphasized that parents should take their time and really nurture all of the relationships involved, including between a woman and her partner (if she has one), the surrogate, and her family (if applicable). She explains, "Surrogacy can be a long and hard road, so be prepared for a marathon. Communication and support is the key to a successful surrogate relationship."

Just like I had with Christine, I felt a kinship with Michelle, and when I asked her whether she felt that there is a great similarity between people who do not or cannot understand her desire to be a gestational carrier and the many people who do not or understand my desire to have another baby after my postpartum depression, she said yes. She empathized that no one on the outside of a story can understand what someone else is going through. She explained that each person has a different journey and that "if you haven't walked in their shoes, you cannot judge their choices!"

In all honesty, if I had the ability to work with a woman like Christine or Michelle or some of the other women I've met with a spirit that is so affectionately generous, gestational carrying would be a difficult option to turn down. And if the gestational carrier wanted to keep in touch with our family, I don't think I'd have any problem with that; in fact, I think I would welcome the chance to thank her, forever, for the gift.

I do not long to be pregnant again. I long for a baby.

Ultimately, with the right amount of funds and the right amount of trust, I think that surrogacy (traditional surrogacy or with a gestational carrier) is a beautiful way to expand a family after postpartum depression. While some concerns and steep financial burdens come along with using a gestational carrier, the major concern around a subsequent bout of severe postpartum depression for a former sufferer can be allayed by choosing this option.

As we have learned, sometimes babies grow in your uterus, sometimes they grow in your heart, and sometimes they grow in another woman whose hand you can hold, either literally or figuratively. The child is just as much a part of you, no matter what vessel carries the baby during pregnancy and then, ultimately, brings the baby into this world. Though surrogacy and gestational carrying are much less popular options for expanding families in this country, we are so lucky with the benefit of science and the benevolence of so many women to have them.

A recent photo that Michelle Griffin has shared on Instagram encapsulates, to me, what surrogacy is all about. It is a photo of her belly, now sticking straight out from her like a torpedo, at thirty-six weeks pregnant. In the photo, Michelle cups her belly with her hands and is joined by three other hands, belonging to three other individuals—one other woman and two men. On one side of her belly, there is the hand of her husband, easily identifiable by the presence of a very distinctive tattoo. On the other side, holding both her belly and each other's hands, are the hands of a man and a woman, belonging to the baby's intended parents. The caption reads, "This little guy was made with love, a little bit of science, and with the help of a bonus family. He will only ever know a world where he was wanted, carefully planned, and awaited . . . As if he isn't the luckiest baby ever."

Indeed.

7

❖ ❖

How to Hang the "Closed" Sign: Choosing *Not* to Expand One's Family

It was the winter of 2018, and by dinnertime the sky was very dark and very clear. Things had shifted so that family dinners were now the norm rather than the exception. The kids could stay up later, we were hungry earlier, and, after years of culinary paralysis, I'd begun to cook again. I had always loved cooking, but I could not so much as pick up a frying pan when I was struggling with my postpartum depression, and, like with many things, I'd had a hard time starting again.

At our family dinner each night the four of us would sit around our small, circular kitchen table, and we would do an activity, one that Belle had brought home with her from school:

"Rose, Thorn, and Bud."

We would go around the table and each person would share their rose, thorn, and bud for the day.

The "rose" would represent the best part of the day—or something that made us happy. The "thorn" was the worst part of the day—or what had brought us down or something that was troubling us. The "bud" was representative of something that was to come—the promise of something to look forward to in the future, near or distant, and perhaps my favorite of all.

On this winter night, we each took a turn, naming our rose, thorn, and bud, and because it was a weekend, Kenny and I agreed to let the kids stay up a little later than usual.

They wanted to dance.

The kids scurried into our den, the coziest little room in our house, and we followed them as they put on one of our favorite songs, so slow and soulful. We all danced around, sometimes in a silly way, sometimes just rocking back and forth, when we felt the music deeply. We did the twist, and we shimmied, and we arched our backs and swayed our hips. I carried Beau in my arms, his little legs wrapped around me, and after I swung him once, he chanted, "Again!" on repeat. Kenny twirled Belle under his arm, and she spun herself into his chest and then out again, so expertly.

I cut in, and Kenny held me and leaned me back into a low dip.

It was romantic, and we were all feeling the feels.

Around the middle of the song, I gathered everyone in a circle in the middle of the room. We held hands and continued to move to the beat, but each person would have a chance to showcase his or her best dance move. Beau moved to the center of our circle and flung his arms around, doing a series of ninja-like poses. Upon her turn, Belle shimmied her nimble little body to the floor and did a unique version of (something that somewhat resembled) break dancing, until Beau fully tackled her to ground.

More laughter.

It is in moments like these, when the four of us are together and happy and such a clearly established unit, that my mind starts to work. That ever-present rumbling of indecision that is with me always manages to shimmy in, taking over my thoughts.

"What if this is it?" I ask myself. "This is pretty great. If this is what I have, then I have more than I could have ever imagined."

But before I can feel an ounce of contentment, I then ask, "But will I regret it? Will I look back and wonder? Will the hole always be here?"

And then I snap back to reality and watch Belle and Beau doing the tango and see Kenny stretching his arm out to me. Just as he always has.

"This is good," I say to myself. And I do not just think it, and I do not just say it to myself as a mantra, but I actually *feel* it. I believe it. I know it.

So I take Kenny's arm and dance, with abandon, spinning around, my hands above my head, and letting it all go. Letting the music and the movement and the moment sweep me away.

It is precious love. It is mine. I am lucky. I am more than lucky—I am blessed. I fought for this. I will keep fighting for this. No matter what happens, I know that I have been gifted with a precious love so profound—one that many will never have the privilege of experiencing. It is precious love, and we will keep dancing, the four of us, until we cannot dance anymore. And then we will dance again the next day.

In the exploration of family expansion after postpartum depression, there is another option that is just as viable, and just as deliberate, as going in for an embryo-transfer procedure, creating a book for an adoption agency, or hiring a surrogate: there is the choice not to expand one's family. To many, this may seem like a default option, but it is far from it.

Many mothers make the valid decision to not try to have future children, biological or otherwise, and for many reasons. For some, they feel complete as they are. For others, their reasoning has nothing to do with their postpartum depression but is about a job or finances or other practical, important concerns.

For many brave mothers, the choice to give their child a healthy mother is a better, more sound decision than giving their family another baby. This decision, like any other, is not easy, nor is it found by the trip down any one road. So many paths lead to this choice, and they are all windy and messy and scary and dark and, often, bright. Some are lined with flowers, and some are lined with glass, but the destination is the same.

Being deeply honest, I envy those who know that their family is complete and have no doubts, at all, in their minds. I have friends who feel such a sense of wholeness and are at peace, so deeply, that the thought of another child seems as preposterous as the thought of growing a third arm (though a third arm would absolutely come in handy, and often). I wish I could feel that way (even more than I wish I could grow a third arm). I have learned that there is no magic number at which all people feel "complete" and that whether it is with one child or twelve, until that number is met, it can feel unsettling at best and agonizing at worst.

For some, it is so clear and painless and happy. For others, it is more like the scar from my cesarean section. From my two babies and the two surgeries it took to deliver them, I have a five-inch scar across my lower abdomen. My abdomen was cut open with a sharp scalpel and blunt dissection devices and cauterized to prevent excess bleeding. It was stretched open, held open, and then sewn shut with internal stitches and stapled closed, on the outside, under a thick, white bandage. It went from being bloody and throbbing to red and tender to pink and tingly to what it is now: flesh colored, thick feeling, and ever present. While it is no longer acutely painful, it is always there. I carry it with me wherever I go. That is what it is like to want another baby and then decide to not have one even when you're not so sure. Sometimes, randomly, it feels sore.

Even when you close your own door after having made your own decision, with agency and power, it can still hurt. Wistfulness abounds.

It can also be frightening. Ghosts can appear, shrouded in cloaks, whispering words like *doubt* and *what if* and *regret* and *who* into the air.

But there is another huge unknown that is the thing that holds me back the most: I need to be here for my children—the children whom I love so fiercely and have now—and I do not want anything to take me away from them. I mean this in every sense.

On a fundamental level, I do not want to have pregnancy- or delivery-related complications that make me sick or, in the worst-case scenario, kill me. My doctor had assured me that he would not let me die on the table, but he can only do so much. In my advocacy work, I have been on panels and given presentations with women who nearly lost their lives while giving birth; I have shared the stage with a father and husband whose wife died, tragically, after giving birth to their second son. When he spoke, we all wept.

I do not want to have postpartum depression again, and though I am confident that I would be able to manage it, both clinically and medicinally, and with great support, it would be an unfortunate burden for my children to endure. When Beau was born, Belle was just three and a half years old. She knows I had postpartum depression, but she does not remember it. She was spared from the darkness. Beau has not known me any other way. But my children are so much older now, and they are empaths and insightful, and if I had postpartum depression, we would not be able to hide it. They have already had to worry about me more than many other children have had to worry about their mothers, and I wince at the thought of adding to their anxieties.

And on a much more benign level, I want to be here for my kids as an involved parent, here to meet their daily needs in the way that I already struggle to do now. I do not find the logistics of motherhood challenging, as Belle and Beau are relatively self-sufficient and their closeness gives me plenty of time to myself. Their activities still coincide, they go to the same school, and Kenny and I are involved parents who show up for school functions and oversee Belle's homework and meet with counselors and teachers and show them endless amounts of love.

With a new baby, by design I would have less time for Belle and Beau, and this scares me as well. In some ways, it feels manageable to me, as they are both in school from 8:30 A.M. until 3 P.M., and so I would only have to manage three kids at once in the morning and after school, before dinnertime. Could I do it? I'm sure I could. Would I be able to be the best mother ever? No. Am I the best mother ever *now*? No. But would I be a better mother to them if I did not have another baby? That is the question. Another baby would signify a level of physical health that I have not experienced in years; perhaps I would be less burdened by my current woes and would be more present, instead of lost in my thoughts, as I so often am.

I would have to learn to add another ball to my juggling act. Just when I've gotten a handle on the two balls, I would have to add a third to the mix.

And this is why at times when we're really happy, or at times when we're mired by deep turmoil, I feel confident that our family is as complete as it will ever be.

I feel secure that I do not need any more happiness, and I feel relieved when I feel as though I could not handle any more difficulty.

More and more, as each day passes and as I get older and as they get older, I feel as though our family is solidifying in a way that would make another baby harder.

They are—we are—my "rose," as our little unit makes me happier than I ever could have imagined. I am grateful for family dinners and dance parties and laughter that makes our bellies hurt.

My "thorn" is the hole—the pain, the indecision. The "hard story" that makes this an issue in the first place. The "why me?" question that I hate to ask but do nonetheless.

My "bud" is every tomorrow. Baby or not. I do not take a single one for granted.

And so, despite the pain, I know that I could close my own door and have the control to do so myself. I could hang the "Closed" sign exactly how I want to and not have the door barricaded for me with a paper reading "Condemned" pinned hastily to the wood.

If my shop is closed, that is for me to decide. And if I close that door, it will be with nothing less than tremendous gratitude, an immense amount of thought, and, most of all, precious, precious love.

Though so many women struggle to make the decision about family expansion after postpartum mood disorders, there are others who are so resolved and so brave that their wisdom astounds me. Here one such woman shares her story about why she decided that her daughter needed a healthy mother and why she herself deserved a healthy life more than anyone needed a new baby.

MELISSA, THIRTY-NINE YEARS OLD

My years of working with the most medically fragile children in the country, and possibly the world, gave me great pause when it came to contemplating the notion of parenthood. My husband and I had discussed having a child at length, countless times. We were told, repeatedly, by "well-intentioned" people, that there was "never a right time to have a baby" as a way to encourage us to make the jump. Maybe so, but I can tell you that there are plenty of wrong times to have a baby.

I can also tell you that not everyone needs to procreate to have a full life.

And so we continued on as the dynamic duo while the parenting conversations took a back seat. We went to Thailand, and we gutted our kitchen. We bought a house, adopted a dog, accelerated our careers, and made great memories with close friends and family.

Once we decided that we did not want to fast-forward ten years and wonder "what if?" our decision was made: we would try to have a baby.

As a medical professional, I knew too much and not enough. I told myself that whether we became parents was no big deal. I think I was protecting my heart from the impending doom of infertility I felt I deserved for not ever having a case of "baby fever," as if that were some sort of qualifier or rite of passage. What is that, anyway? Besides, we'd been happy together for years; it was no big deal, right? You can't miss what you don't have.

And so it was hard to get pregnant. It was also sort of weird when we went to the reproductive endocrinologist. I mean, I wanted to know that I could get pregnant and carry a baby to term, but I certainly was not ready for that man (a man other than my husband) to impregnate me by way of modern medicine. I guess you could say my husband and I were lukewarm about procreating, but we wanted the option. We certainly were not typical RE (reproductive endocrinology) patients. Of course, being science nerds, we asked lots of great questions. We knew what next steps were available if we chose them. Instead, we decided to plan a trip that would be either a "babymoon" if I ultimately got pregnant or the first of many annual international trips if we could not conceive.

Our baby was present when our hot-air balloon made a surprise landing in Cappadocia, Turkey, many months later. We had gotten pregnant on our own after a hysterosalpinogram (an uncomfortable test that involves injecting dye into the fallopian tubes to assess their viability and check for any blockages) and a dash of some fabulous acupuncture. We just didn't know it yet.

Newsflash: If you're trying to get pregnant and it's taking longer than you think it should, you will be surrounded by more pregnant people than you thought possible, and regularly. Did I mention that I was a pediatric nurse, on a unit full of women of childbearing age at the time? It was a strange dynamic in which no one spoke of infertility or postpartum struggles, period, until you piped up, at which point, like the flip of a switch, the floodgates would open. Once I shared my story, everyone else on the unit started sharing their stories, and the sheer number of women with stories of infertility was immense. I learned this when I was early into my pregnancy and sharing how happily cautious I was. Then I would hear the stories of colleagues and friends who had quietly suffered miscarriages or had moved out of state to have their IVF covered by insurance. The same type of wordfall happened when I started speaking about postpartum maternal health and admitted that every day was not a trip to the unicorn forest.

It seemed as though as soon as women become mothers, or even thought of it, they took this silent oath. We've been trained to just share the rainbows and butterflies. What about the miscarriages? What about the leaking breasts or the popped cesarean-section sutures? Why was everyone around me silently stepping on Legos and forcing themselves to be superhuman as if their lives had not just been flipped upside down? I would not perpetuate the myths.

I never had strangers rub my belly—thank goodness for that. I did get the eye rolls and the passive aggressive "Oh, I could never do that—I like to plan, blah, blah," whenever I'd announce we weren't going to learn our growing fetus's gender. People didn't get it, but they didn't have to. I worked in the cardiac intensive-care unit at a children's hospital. I wanted to know that my baby had four chambers in their heart. I gave zero fucks about a penis or a vagina. Despite this, or because of this, I must note that while I did not give any fucks, I was prepared as fuck. Like, as prepared as you can be when you are hypothetically raising a child you have not ever met. I was a married career woman–homeowner who chose pregnancy. I had peed on so many ovulation sticks waiting for the smiley face to know when I could get pregnant. I had boys' and girls' clothes ready, thanks to my sister, Joanna. Oh, and get this: my husband and I actually got along really well.

Because life works out in the strangest of ways, when I was twenty-three weeks pregnant, my husband had a biopsy done of a lymph node on his neck. I was in the waiting room, drinking hot tea, which was one of my favorite pastimes, hoping his surgeon and anesthesiologists were on their A game. The open-neck biopsy went fabulously well. It was all good.

Until it wasn't. Three weeks later, when we went in for our follow-up, we walked into the doctor's office prepared to talk about how nonexistent his scar was. Good job, Mister Plastic-Surgery ENT (ear, nose, and throat) Combo Doctor! Rock on.

But before I started with the high fives, I was stopped in my tracks. My memory is blurry, but I know that the man wore a white coat. He said the words *cancer* and *oncologist* and *lymphoma* and . . . the world went black. I was twenty-six weeks pregnant, in the fetal position, on a bathroom floor in the doctor's office, with snot running down my face when Chris picked me up. What the fuck had just happened to our world? All of our deliberate planning? Our zen?

His chemotherapy was scheduled initially for the day after our baby shower. My husband, who never had the cold or flu in the five years since I'd known him, decided to jump straight to cancer for his first marital illness. Spoiler: He's now okay. But for a decent amount of time, he wasn't. Neither was I. We were not okay at all. We also suffered from the uncommon affliction known as always-being-incredibly-strong-and-having-our-acts-together, so the list of people who jumped to help us was rather small—but, thankfully, mighty. Never stop checking on your strong friends.

I had to cope with so many things at once: I was a wife and a caretaker, a pregnant woman and a nurse. These things were hard to reconcile. At the baby's anatomy scan, a detailed ultrasound during which time you can find out whether the baby is a boy or a girl, I braced for news that would not involve what was between my fetus's legs. People continued to tell me that I would not be given a situation that I couldn't handle. This is not reassuring for a pediatric nurse. This made me scared that I would have a critically ill child. First I thought I wouldn't be able to get pregnant as punishment for never having had baby fever. Now I was deeply afraid my child would be sick. I have seen the greatest love between parents and children whether healthy or sick. I have also seen families struggle, torn apart, watching their tiny humans get poked and prodded. I knew I was strong. I know I am strong. If this is what parenthood would be for us, if it would tear our marriage apart, if it would cause me to see my fragile child ache regularly, I just couldn't do it.

With great relief, at our anatomy scan I learned then that there were four chambers of the baby's heart, skin over the spine, beautiful lungs forming; all of the parts were growing as expected for a healthy baby. I went out that night for dinner with my sister and sister-in-law and celebrated.

Nothing says "healthy baby" like mushroom soup in a shot glass at one of my favorite restaurants. The next day I pulled the trigger on the nursery furniture, which I learned needs as much lead time as a wedding dress. Of note, the collection is called "Belize," which happens to be where we honeymooned. Yep, I am a total sap.

A relief fell over me after that ultrasound. My husband's surgery was three weeks later. Mathematically speaking, then, I had three weeks of pregnancy when I was *not* worried. The baby was healthy (hooray!), and the baby daddy was not. My husband felt great and looked as healthy as could be. Our second opinion led us to another medical institution that changed his treatment plan to watch and wait. This was so hard. We had spent the previous fifteen days learning about the chemotherapy that he would need and were basically begging for it to begin. So to watch and wait did not seem like a superior option. Although we did just that. (Fast-forward, and we watched and waited until he was then later treated for non-Hodgkin's lymphoma with Epstein-Barr virus. Our daughter was eighteen months old when the treatments began. They lasted for about eight months. We didn't realize it then, because it was incredibly difficult, but had we experienced chemo earlier on in her life, it would have been impossible to bear.)

I loved being pregnant. I felt amazing. I worked incredibly long shifts, making some days difficult, but, overall, pregnancy was my jam. I felt beautiful and peaceful and terrified. Once my husband was diagnosed with cancer, my feelings were so all over the place. This was when I really learned that you could be incredibly happy about one thing and devastated by another all at once. To say we were on a roller coaster would be a gross understatement. In my mind, I had convinced myself that my baby was a boy and that he would grow up protecting his momma and that my husband would die, soon. Anxiety makes us believe things so deeply, and fear disguises itself as intuition. Thankfully, I am not always right.

Being a nurse and a realist, I refused to have a birth plan. What I did have was a short list of what I did not want, and knew the baby called the shots on most everything else. On my list of no-thank-you items: induction and C-section. I didn't care who performed the delivery, just as long as my nurse was awesome, since the nurse is the one with you for twelve hours at a time. I was not worried about if there were music playing, and I was completely open to pain management or not. My C-section didn't happen until after pushing for three hours and twenty minutes. This was about eighteen hours after my induction.

Yep—welcome to motherhood, you tired, exhausted, shaky girl. Get used to being really flexible.

Welcome, Harper Rose Bocage. My daughter.

We started breastfeeding right away. Harper knew what to do, and, apparently, I did too. I was induced for potential IUGR (intrauterine growth restriction). I wanted to refuse the induction, but if the placenta stopped working, I did not want to risk anything. The catch-22 choices started even before my daughter and I had ever even met. "Baby Bocage" would show this type A, fun-loving momma that even the best plans can erupt. IUGR she was not, and let me just tell you, my breast milk must have been chock-full of calories, because my girl plumped up, and fast.

On the list of things I could control: breastfeeding. I could feed my baby and watch her grow. I knew I'd try to breastfeed, but I didn't know just how much it would mean to me. Thankfully, for us it was easy. I took care of her with such precision. I kept a journal for ten weeks, where I documented every feed, stating which breast, and how many minutes she nursed. I documented every diaper change. I was a critical-care nurse, so all of this documenting was pretty natural for me. What I learned was that a baby fed by mouth, on demand, was way different from the babies I was tube feeding every three hours at the hospital.

Leading up to my six-week postpartum appointment, I knew that I was anxious—really anxious. My husband insisted on taking me to this appointment, so I knew he'd seen a change in me too. I was so worried about returning to work. I did not want to leave my daughter. I also did not want to take care of babies that would die. Sometimes when our little girl was sleeping, I'd wake her or make her stir to know she was okay. I'd listen to her heart rate or count her respirations to make sure she was safe. I wouldn't let her sleep anywhere but next to me. Her nursery was beautiful and ready before she came home, but she'd never end up sleeping even a night in there until she was six months old. I thought she'd die of SIDS (sudden infant death syndrome). I was afraid the nurse in me would miss something obvious and I would later regret her suffering for my stupidity. How much of this was sleep deprivation, how much of this was real-life occupational hazard, and how much of this was my hormones? Harper is six years old now, and I still don't know how to slice up what caused what.

My physician let me talk for all of five minutes before she said, "Look, Melissa. You haven't made eye contact with me since you walked in the office, you're not going back to work, and you need to see a psychiatrist and psychologist before going back to your life."

I was so relieved. I would see whomever the heck she wanted me to if it kept me out of work. I could not leave my baby. I had to take care of her. I was so lost. My husband was amazing. "A hands-on dad," some people said. Those people made me chuckle and also made me angry because, duh, he's a dad, so all hands had better be on.

That being said, I felt alone. I had to take care of the baby. I had to. I had to keep my intake and output journal. I had to go talk to someone about my feelings. Looking back, I guess with a cancer diagnosis during pregnancy, on top of paradigm shifts and sleep-pattern changes at home, it would be shocking if I didn't have postpartum depression and postpartum anxiety. And after having worked in labor and delivery, I also now think it would be shocking if the delivery of my first and only child had actually gone as I'd imagined. I found myself incredibly crushed, too, when realizing my expectations of others were far higher than they were willing to reach. For years others had encouraged us to have a baby, but when the reality happened, we learned that what we really had was each other.

Please do not get me wrong: During that first year postpartum, if my husband had sent me an au pair and never come home, I would have been fine with that. I still am not certain if that's a new-momma thing or a postpartum thing. But it is the truth. But like everything else, we found a new normal, and that we-get-along thing I mentioned before? Well, we still do.

Life at home with a newborn was interesting. If you wanted me to brush my teeth, eat lunch, and take care of the baby, I would have said, "Oh, hell no." All I could do was take care of her. As for me, I'm sure I must have showered here and there. I also had nice pajamas. I had a new wardrobe of easy boob-removal tops. I basically turned myself into a milking shell. We did start going to baby music classes once a week when she was six weeks. This was great, but I swear it would take me all week to mentally prepare for gathering up all the baby gear and going the next week. But each week I'd talk to the other moms more and more. Finally, we all admitted we had no freakin' clue what we were doing. Our baby-shaped blobs lay on the floor as we enticed them with music. Getting out of the house was so necessary.

Spending so much time at home without my husband, my other half, my everyday friend for seven years before we'd created a human, was hard and was weird and was lonely. This was especially difficult since I let the expectations I'd had for others begin to eat away at me. Straight away I started to stress about having an only child. You had to have two; you just had to—that's what was normal, what was expected. Besides, I loved being pregnant. Yes, my daughter's delivery had been a disaster, but who was I to keep my precious daughter from the joy of a sibling?

But fast-forward a couple of years, and I have learned that I am not everyone and I am not governed by one finite set of rules. Who I am is me. And *me* is the best parenting decision that I ever made. Also, I have learned there is no normal and there are no rules. It took a while, but once I learned this, it stuck. Besides, a sibling is not nearly even close to the only joy you can offer a child, and realistically, a sibling is not always a joy.

Due to the postpartum anxiety and depression I suffered, my husband's cancer and chemo, and an unfortunate fall I took down some stairs, I did not feel like myself at least until Harper was four years old. I revisited the idea of another child so many times. I was in a bunch of "one and only" Facebook groups that only served to make me want to have more kids just to prove some of those judgmental women wrong. I didn't have any weird or ill feelings toward others who had multiple children. I just didn't identify with them. Not when she was six months, eighteen months, three years, or, even now, six years old. I could not parent another child as much as I've parented Harper. The mom guilt alone would probably kill me. Besides, how much sense would it really make to jeopardize my health to make another tiny human? Children are not collector's items.

I also kept the pledge I'd made while pregnant when I'd promised myself and others that I would not lie through life, making myself feel better and others feel worse. I saw so many women around me talking about the joys of motherhood, and I understood it and also resented the misrepresentation. I *did not* perpetuate the myth. I wish I could say that this is where the facade related to parenting ended, but I would be doing a great disservice. I was stopped in my tracks when I first saw the video of another mental-health sufferer on YouTube. Alexis Joy D'Achille's memorial YouTube video popped up on my Facebook feed, and I learned of the tragic story of a woman who, like me, had one daughter and suffered from postpartum depression, but who, unlike me, lost her battle. While staring at the Facebook video, and watching it on repeat, I saw her—really saw her—and while I was never suicidal, I saw myself. I knew then that my voice was strong, my heart was ready, and *my* Legos were not going to be stepped on in silence.

My husband and I talked about growing our family and about not growing our family, many times. We both felt complete with our daughter, but we did toss around the idea of more children. He knew that for a while there I was tortured, in that I wanted to want more kids. But I didn't *actually* want more kids. I felt so weird that the "baby fever" that "everyone" had (and, P.S., this is a myth!) was lost on me. Admitting that I wanted to want more kids sounds crazy to me now. You cannot want to want anything. It's silly. Trying to be more or less of someone to appeal to others is the last parenting technique I'd ever recommend.

Family size is such a personal choice. It is not a decision to be made lightly. Although often it is a decision that you cannot make on your own. For a long time, I think both my husband and I thought that if I accidentally got pregnant, then we'd have an answer. That sparked the realest talk of my life when I finally admitted to myself, and to him, that another pregnancy, delivery, and postpartum period would ruin me and destroy the family we'd fought so hard to create. In my mind our daughter had almost lost her father already; she was not going to ever risk losing me—not if I could help it.

I sobbed. I sobbed in his arms. I snotted on his sleeve. Marriage is so glamorous.

"We won't figure it out," I said. "I don't want to figure it out. If we have another baby, we need to probably move. I don't want to move. We would need to change our daughter's school, and I don't want to change that." We listed all of the things that would need to change, and despite the fact that we are flexible people, and capable of adapting to change, something welled up inside of me. Well, it was more of an emotional volcano that erupted.

"*Me*," I said to my husband. "*Me*. I cannot lose *me* again. I just can't. My mental health cannot chance the hit of a baby." Sometimes the things are the hardest to admit are the most helpful at the same time.

Yes, I loved being pregnant. I love being a mom more than everything. But when I think of another baby and all of the changes, perceived and real, I immediately think of all that our family would lose. I need to be there to see Harper at gymnastics and not be chasing a baby. I need to work. I need to stay at my job, where I feel like my brain and compassion help others. I even shared with my husband that I need to be his wife and that if I were to accidentally get pregnant, I think I'd want an immediate divorce, since I would somehow find a way to blame him.

"I need to be me."

Self-care is not indulgent; it is necessary. And a wise friend once told me that she felt finished having children after her third, that I felt finished after my first, and that neither is right or wrong, just different.

When I came to the realization in my heart that another baby would most certainly send me spiraling downward mentally, I began to distance myself from my husband. While we knew we were "one and done," he had not yet had a vasectomy, and I began to view him as a penis full of babies. I had finally admitted the devastation I would feel for him, our daughter, and myself if I ever became pregnant again. I surprised him, I shocked myself, and within six months he was at the urologist on his own account. He made the appointment. He knew our choice, and he knew how lost I'd become if that choice were ever taken from us. And once again he protected me, and he protected our family, and I fell in love with him all over again. Our daughter was given the most joyous gift of a lifetime to make memories within a stable, loving, fun, happy home.

What I've learned and know to be true deep in my soul is that I want my daughter to have her independence, her carefree, questioning spirit, and her role model emulating what *living* looks like. I want my daughter to be the remarkable human she is—like me, a total sap, and so with us, my husband is surrounded by glitter and smiles.

I believe if I had another kiddo, I'd be much better at it. I already had a trial run. That being said, instead, I choose us.

I choose us, all day, every day.

The three of us and our dog—we're our family. We all just fit. I believe the ability to adapt is very important and that there are times when we have to live in survival mode. One day I just realized that I would *not* demonstrate that as my baseline behavior. After all, I have a little girl looking up to me, and merely surviving just will not do, even when it's hard; thriving is the goal.

I quit those "one and only" Facebook groups and made my own group. I'm still taken aback when I realize there are over four hundred members locally now. I'm not weird. It's not just me who has an only child. There are some families who have lost a spouse, some parents who have struggled with infertility, and some who are uncertain whether they're finished having children. When I started talking, they started talking back. Parenting has taught me, from the very first time we seriously chose to begin to try to become pregnant, that we are all more the same than we are different. When we speak up, when we use our voices, when we validate others and share our experiences, we permit happiness. My daughter has so much joy, and now she has parents who know what that truly means.

If you're lucky enough to realize that life is full of choices, you can also empower yourself to make them for the right reasons. It takes bravery, but we are brave.

So what does life look today? Our house is full of joy and laughter. I make frequent enough inappropriate comments that my husband likely does feel as if he has two children at times, all the while grateful that his wife has started laughing again and hasn't stopped. My daughter and I dance, research, read, play, and explore. My husband and I laugh and support one another. We show our daughter what mutual respect looks like. We take turns having one-on-one time with her so we can fill our own cups too. Our family will never grow in size by number of children, but it will continue to flourish in all other ways. I have never been more proud to share choices that have made our home and lives bright. I am thrilled to see and experience our daughter's childhood years together, stronger than ever before, and, gosh, that one child of ours just *wows* me. I now know and trust that our child(ren) will shine independently of every decision we make. We should always remember to give them the credit and the cheering that they deserve. They are so much more than their family spot.

With lots of love, light, and a holiday vasectomy wish granted in Philadelphia, Melissa

8

When You Leave the Door Ajar, the Weather Is Always Windy: You Just Aren't Sure

There is a place that exists in between "my shop is closed" and "wide open for business," and it is the hardest place for me to be. Though conventional wisdom would likely lead people to believe that the "maybe baby" place is happier than the "no baby" place, because in it there is hope, it feels more like limbo. It is like being a human wishbone, waiting to see which side of you will win the contest when you finally crack in half.

In this middle place, I do not have a door firmly closed from which I can walk away. I do not get to lock this door or put any distance between myself and the shop I carry within me. In this middle place, I do not have a clearly happy future, I do not have any peace, I do not have a baby; I have opacity and angst.

While my shop is no longer closed, it has a faulty door hinge, and so it swings open with any gust of wind or even the slightest breeze. The sound of the door opening and then slamming shut on repeat is deafening. It gives me a perpetual headache. The whoosh of the gusty air on my skin gives me windburn, and so I am always raw. The sign in the window has been taken down; it does not read *open*, nor does it read *closed*, and that confuses everyone. People pop in, awkwardly, and do not know exactly what to say to me when they see me there, with an unlocked, swinging door but no clear sense of the shop's status.

Some lights are on, and others are off. Some shelves are stocked, and others are bare. In many ways, it is a sad shop to visit. It is trying so hard—too hard—and yet missing the mark. The store is not successful, because it keeps odd hours and is unpredictable. The lights flicker. Everything seems ephemeral.

I hate the middle place, but the middle place is where I call home.

I do not think that I could possibly overstate the amount of mental energy I expend on the topic of another baby. It is with me all the time, like an appendage. Or a tattoo. In fact, I have even seriously thought about getting a tattoo to symbolize this third child, whether the child manifests or not, just to honor its weight in my heart. I actually got each of my other three tattoos after having survived postpartum depression, and I have worn them like badges of honor—strength. Growing up, I never thought I would get inked, and I'm grateful that these permanent adornments were done deliberately rather than, say, having gotten a hasty symbol on my lower back after a high school graduation party. I am not the "hasty huge permanent decision" type, if I have yet to make that clear.

I made sure that each one of my tattoos was discreet and, most important, something that I never would—never could—regret. My first tattoo, done the week before I turned twenty-nine, is my signature of my maiden name: Fox. It is on my right side, on my rib cage. To me, it symbolizes my fortitude and is the last name of my angels.

My second tattoo is of the words *belle et beau*, written in the lowercase script of a dear friend. This tattoo is on the exact same spot as my first, but on the left side; it is the spot closest to my heart. While the words are in French, and translate to "beautiful and handsome," they are the names of my two children—the individuals who make my heart beat each day.

My third tattoo (located on a part of my body for which I do not know the name, so I just call it my right-lower-outside-next-to-side-boob-area-part-of-my-shoulder-blade) is the word *jolie*, French for "pretty," a nickname given to me by my Poppop since birth, and something I will cherish, always.

To get a tattoo to symbolize my desire for a third child seems both empowering and, in some ways, bleak. Since it would be permanently written on my body, I want to make sure that the ink that would be placed within me would be healing and not hurtful. I need to know that it would be a sentimental tribute and not a sorrowful reminder only serving to perpetuate my pain.

In thinking about a new symbol to place permanently on my body—one that would feel appropriate and meaningful and moving and right—I have come back to the one thing I know best: words. My idea for a fourth tattoo is the word *trace* in tiny letters, to be written in a spot that is also close to my heart. I like the word as a stand-alone, as I think it is evocative and artistic and, perhaps, sexy. Fingertips tracing the lines and swirls and imperfections. But it is also a play on words. *Tres*, in Spanish, means "three," and it would be my surreptitious homage to the number that means so much to me.

Like a tattoo, this internal battle is under my skin and is always there, waging war within me all day, every day.

Over the years, this topic comes up, even when I do not ask for it to be raised. And when I explain my situation, in short form—or, more often, in great detail (read: oversharing)—there is an idea that has been floated to me not a few times. It is the notion that perhaps my desperation for another baby is because I was told that I cannot have one and that this lack of control is what is fueling my longing more than the actual desire to add a third child to our family. The premise is not completely flawed; I think that a lot of my behaviors can be attributed to the pursuit of obtaining more control than I (or any of us, really) has in this life. I could never describe myself as being zen, nor am I someone who can accept the reality of any situation and say, "It is what it is," as I would be lying, and if I did not like something, I would try to fix it.

But in this case, when I have searched my soul for answers, I do not think that I want a baby just because someone told me that I cannot have one. Not even a little bit. I understand how we are predisposed to wanting the proverbial forbidden fruit, but in this case, the notion does not resonate.

Recently I was sitting at our small, round, white kitchen table, enjoying Sunday-night dinner with Kenny and the kids. I was drinking water from a giant, glass beer stein emblazoned with the coat of arms and Greek letters of my husband's college fraternity (oh, the irony!) when I sensed the opportunity for a teachable moment. I began explaining the "glass half full" notion to Belle and Beau as a way to teach them about optimism and pessimism.

"It's like if there's a day when the forecast calls for 50 percent rain showers," I explained. "For someone who is optimistic, they might look at that as having a 50 percent chance of a sunny day. For someone who's more pessimistic, they would see it as a 50 percent chance of rain."

I was not sure whether they were getting it, and so I held up my giant glass for them, in which the water line was at the exact halfway point between the top and bottom.

"Do you see this here? You might hear people talk about someone being 'glass half full,' and that means that, for that person, who is a more optimistic person, they would look at my water glass and see the water that was in it. They would look at the good. But someone who is a 'glass half empty' person might look at the glass and be grumpy about it because I had already drunk half of the water."

And then, as it often does, my mind started to race.

As Kenny continued the explanation for them, using as examples Eeyore and Piglet, from *Winnie-the-Pooh*, I started to turn the "glass half full" metaphor on its head, as it swirled around in *my* head.

"But let's say it's something that you really don't want to drink," I posited. "Let's say the glass is filled to the top, and then seeing it halfway finished is actually a relief. What about then?"

I thought, queasily, of the times that I've had to hold my nose and choke down a chalky, repellent barium drink before a computed-tomography scan. Or the cloying orange bottle of liquid glucose before the gestational-diabetes screenings during pregnancy. Or a glass of oaky chardonnay.

"In those instances, having the glass empty would actually be the happy, optimistic thought!"

Kenny shook his head, playfully, at how our light dinner conversation had taken this deep, philosophical turn.

It occurred to me then that this is just like the baby decision: everyone looks at the world differently, and people are dynamic, as lives evolve. Having more can feel like less, less can feel like more, full can feel empty, and emptiness can feel whole. It's all about perspective.

Beau then made a dessert of cookie dough sandwiched between two Oreo cookies, and I couldn't help but laugh. I wouldn't be deciding anything that night, but as I thought about the picture of our family, I felt grateful, with that "cup runneth over" feeling, though I knew that as the night went on my thoughts would continue to shift and morph and change, as they always do.

So in that moment, I decided that the best I could do was to bite into a piece of raw cookie dough and hope for the best.

The middle place is a lonely, uncomfortable place to be. Like that half-way place in a glass of water, there is no clear answer to be found in the middle place. The door opens, the door closes, and with each swing of the solid, wooden frame, I shudder or shiver or crawl behind my shop's counter to cry. I trace the lines on my stomach, once condemned as a "teardown," now flat and covered in shallow tunnels that resemble stretch marks. I trace the shape of what I am and mentally outline the life I think I should have, and the lights flicker around me, and the door slams as a gust of wind whips at my fragile skin, as I look for the door sign and try not to break as I go.

I know that I am not alone in the middle place. This brings me relief and also pain. I do not want others to live with the suffocating indecision that plagues me daily, but I know that this is the reality of so many. In this chapter, four people courageously, eloquently, exquisitely share their stories, in their own words, about the agony of indecision and how it informs so much of our lives—past, present, and future.

Three incredible women write about their journeys with severe perinatal distress.

And, for the first time, there are the words of a man.

He writes in the first person. He shares his experience candidly, beautifully, and breathtakingly.

He is my husband, Kenny, and his voice should be heard.

BECKY, FORTY-THREE YEARS OLD

There was a knock on the door. Again. It seemed to happen at least once an hour; in the three days since I had given birth, my hospital room had become a revolving door, with staff coming in and out endlessly. This time it was a social worker.

"Has anyone talked with you about postpartum depression?" she asked.

I quickly scanned my brain. It was hard to remember much of anything, as the lack of sleep and information overload had taken its toll. I recalled the lactation consultant and her lessons on proper latch technique, the ten minutes someone spent talking about how to swaddle my son, when to use the bulb aspirator. But I couldn't recall any talk of postpartum depression.

"I know what it is," I answered. "But I don't think we discussed it with anyone since I've been here. It's just depression after the baby is born, right? Hormones?"

"Kind of," she answered with a gentle smile. "You just need to pay close attention to your thoughts and feelings. If any seem out of the ordinary, contact your doctor immediately."

I smirked. I hadn't felt "normal" since the day I'd seen two lines on a plastic stick in my bathroom. How would I know what normal was ever again?

I accepted the brochure from her outstretched hand, and my husband filed it away among all the other papers we had been given. The width of our stack was hovering around cinder block–size, and I couldn't guess what was in there if you'd paid me.

That was my education on postpartum depression.

Our first few days at home were a blur. I existed in a daze, created by a combination of exhaustion and anxiety. Fortunately, my son was nursing like a champ. But my breasts had turned to granite, and his latch felt like I was inserting my nipple into a pencil sharpener. One that had been lubed up with acid. I assumed this was normal and carried on as best I could.

I can't say I was happy. I loved my son, but I felt like I'd been imprisoned in a nursery and would live on an endless conveyor belt of breastfeeding, burping, changing diapers, and tears. "But," I'd tell myself, "women have been doing this for centuries. This must be normal. My resistance must be because I'm not a good mother."

After about a week at home, my husband told me his father and step-mother would be coming over to meet our son. My reaction was physical. My stomach felt like I'd just ascended a massive loop on a roller coaster, and my palms were slick with sweat.

"He's too little to see anyone," I pleaded. "Can they come next week instead?"

"He'll be two weeks old by then," my husband began in a tone I did not like one bit. "Besides, your parents have been here since the day he was born, and you've had no problem with that."

"It's different," I began, before he interrupted me.

"So your family's okay but mine's not?" he asked. I could not tell whether he was angry or hurt. I think it was some mixture of the two.

"I don't know," I said with tears now pooling in the corners of my eyes. "I know it sounds weird, but I'm just not ready."

"It's my dad. It's not a group of strangers. My family deserves to meet him also," he explained. "They'll be here tomorrow at five." With that he walked out of the room and the conversation was finished. He had decided, and the decision was final.

I felt like I was being irrational, and yet I could not make peace with the idea of anyone else holding my son. And he was right: my parents *had* been around since the night before the birth. Why did this feel differ-ent? I decided that I was being irrational and, therefore, was obviously ill equipped to be a mother.

That was the first time I attacked myself. Or, rather, the first time I let my brain tell me things that were not true.

Over the next twenty-four hours I embarked upon my first postpartum downward spiral. I could not piece together the puzzle—explanations for my foreign feelings and reactions—and it sent me on a journey to nowhere. Like a maze with no way out. I wanted to understand why I was so afraid of visitors meeting my son, but I had no logical reasons. So I improvised my answers.

You're a bad mom. You shouldn't have had a baby. Your husband and son would be better off without you.

I begged my husband to pack up the baby and depart for his mother's house. It made the most sense to me. I clearly couldn't be a mother, and I felt what I was sure was his silent judgment burning a hole in my heart.

He told me I was being ridiculous. "You're tired," he explained. "No," I thought. "I'm a bad person."

Later that day I had a flash of clarity. Was this postpartum depression, I wondered? I thought back to the brochure we'd been given and went to find it in the pile of hospital paperwork cluttering our kitchen countertop.

I shuffled through the documents until I found it. I quickly scanned it, looking for anything that resembled what I'd been feeling. Yet nothing I read was familiar, so I ruled out postpartum depression and came back to my original "bad mom" diagnosis. It turns out my instincts were correct; I just didn't have the proper help to diagnose it in time. I was indeed suffering from postpartum depression, a small cloud that would soon grow into complete darkness that would block out the sunshine and take over my life.

I just didn't know it at the time.

Over the next few months I vacillated between wanting to run away and taking my own life. I had plans for both. To run away, I would simply hightail it to the park down the street and go to sleep. A bench or the ground would do. And when the police showed up to question the crazy lady, I'd pretend I was a mute. Then, I reasoned, they'd take me to jail, and I could sleep even more. In hindsight, it sounds absolutely delusional. But at the time I thought the plan was flawless.

The more concerning plan was the one to take my life. I need to run an errand, I'd say. Then I would set out in my car and find a wall to drive into. I never told anyone that. While I had it all mapped out in my mind, that's where it stayed. For that I will always be thankful.

I stopped eating—not because I was trying to lose the baby weight. Because I had no appetite. I would shove a lone piece of turkey into my mouth once a day as sustenance so I could at least continue breastfeeding my son. I felt like that was the only thing I was good for and needed to be able to continue giving him that.

With a newborn, sleep is elusive. Yet, when I actually had the opportunity to rest, I couldn't. Insomnia took over. I began cleaning baseboards with Q-tips at 3 A.M., anything to keep busy and stop my mind from talking to me. But I could never silence it entirely. My mind kept up the attacks on repeat.

I am a bad mom, I am a bad person, and I just have to get my son through these first few months, and then I'll leave. If I can last that long.

I didn't ask for help because I was convinced that every new mother felt this way. My inability to handle the norm clearly meant I was a failure. This unendurable situation was something I just had to endure, to suck it up and smile. Speaking out would simply be a burden to anyone forced to listen. So I continued. Feeding, diapering, cleaning in the middle of the night. Forcing a smile and answering "Great!" when anyone asked how I was doing.

My husband and I were drifting apart. Or maybe we just couldn't see each other in the midst of this blinding fog that had enveloped our lives. It was more like tear gas, actually. Painful and attacking. He became the enemy, our son seemingly pitting us against one another. I needed things from my husband that I was unable to express; he didn't know how to help me and grew frustrated when his attempts were met with anger.

I wanted a divorce, I decided. He wasn't the man I'd fallen in love with and married. Again, I would just get my son through a few months of breastfeeding before I did anything. Divorce would mean shared custody, and I didn't want to deprive my child of my milk, I reasoned. Another future plan I filed away in my brain. To be enacted when the time was right.

I held on as best as I could until one day I let go. My son was crying, as babies do. But I couldn't handle it. The wails caused a physical reaction in my body that was like nothing I'd ever felt. I wanted to scratch my skin and pull out my hair. I tried to soothe him to no avail. I placed him down in his bassinet and walked into my kitchen, where I grabbed the first thing I saw, a plastic cup, and hurled it against the wall. I fell to the ground sobbing.

"I give up, I give up!" I screamed. To everyone and no one. "Please," I begged of God and the universe. "Help me be a mother. I don't know how."

My son and I cried in unison for about a minute, though it felt like much longer. I then crawled on my hands and knees to where I had dropped my cell phone earlier and called my husband at work.

"Please come home now," I said in a calm voice that felt foreign after my outburst. "I need help."

He came home, and I drove straight to my OBGYN's office. I walked in, and, as soon as the office manager saw me, she walked wordlessly toward me and enveloped me in a hug. I sobbed, and she held me in that moment when I was unable to stand on my own.

She escorted me to an exam room and sat me down. My favorite nurse, the one who had seen me through all those exams and twice-weekly non-stress tests during my pregnancy, soon appeared bearing a plate of pumpkin bread. "Eat," she instructed. And I did. I was suddenly ravenous; the dam broke, and I was able to accept help in every form.

I was there for a while. My doctor assessed me and decided I was not going to harm myself or anyone else. I answered questions, speaking honestly about the previous few months. I heard the words *postpartum depression.* "Yes, I want to try medication," I answered when asked.

I was prescribed Zoloft, and we created a plan. I talked with my husband, and my parents stopped their lives to come and stay with us so I wouldn't be alone during the day. I was going to get better, I was told, but I couldn't do it alone. And I didn't need to try.

While that day was the beginning of my healing, it was far from the beginning of the end, I would soon learn.

The medication helped tremendously. Within two weeks I saw the old me in the mirror. It was still a bit hazy, as if the steam from a shower were clouding my view, But she was there. I hadn't realized how much I'd missed her until that moment.

I began seeing a therapist. Shared my story with family, friends, and even strangers on social media. I was shocked at how many women had gone through the same thing I had. It made me feel less alone, but I was also angry. Why wasn't this talked about more? If I had known my feelings weren't normal, would I have sought help sooner? I thought of all the time I'd lost with my son. Months of going through the motions, willing time to pass. Not being able to enjoy him.

The next year was full of ups and downs. I felt better, overall. Smiled real and true smiles. Loved my child and was fully present in each moment of his life. All the aspects of motherhood that had eluded me were now part of my daily life, and I was thankful.

I had setbacks. But I knew the signs, what to look for and, most important, what to do. I used my voice and was honest about my feelings. My medication was changed a few times. Increased, actually, but I never cared. I was always happy that something existed that could help. That made me whole again and helped me ignore the lies my mind told me. I knew I was a good mother.

Once that fog cleared, my husband and I found our way back to one another. Emotionally and physically. Yet we were quick to silence anyone who asked about the possibility of a second child. "We're one and done," we'd say, almost robotically. It was our canned response.

But we believed it. Neither of us felt like we were sacrificing our past dreams of having a large family. After all, we'd been able to conceive naturally a few months after my fortieth birthday. We knew how lucky we were. Given our age and my experience with PPD, we felt no need to press our luck and try again.

Looking back, I'm not sure if we really felt that way or if we were just saying that because we believed we should. It was beyond my PPD; I didn't want to tempt fate. We already had a healthy baby. I worried I was selfish for wanting more.

We had initially been protected by time—for a short while, at least. In the very beginning, no one had asked, or expected, us to be thinking about having another baby for the first six, nine months. But it was somewhere around our son's first birthday that the invisible shield of protection faltered and the questions started coming. At his birthday party, in fact.

My husband's cousin, a childless man in his late thirties, asked it, as we were all gathered around my son, watching him stick his entire face into a cake that was frosted to look like a cheeseburger.

"When are you two going to get to work on a brother or sister for him?" He was smiling at his own question. "You know you don't have much time left." He laughed and looked around, as if proud of himself for knowing my age (forty-two at the time).

We quickly dismissed him, saying something about how we hadn't even thought about it yet. But it didn't matter: the veil had been lifted, and the question was now conspicuous. Sitting there, staring at us. Waiting for our decision.

We never discussed it beyond one of us saying "We can't" and the other nodding in agreement. Which is odd, in hindsight, because my husband and I tend to overanalyze what to eat for breakfast. Not *this* massive, important decision, however. This was different. We just ignored it and pretended it wasn't the flashing red light it had become.

Not making a decision was the easy way out. We were saying no while not actually doing anything. Our ambivalence and indecision was our answer. There would be no second baby.

The first time I felt an inkling of doubt about our "no" was when a friend announced her second pregnancy. Her son was around the same age as mine, and the news hit me like a truck. Procrastinating on making a decision had been fueled, partly, by my belief that my son was still too young for us to even entertain the notion of a second pregnancy.

That reasoning—or excuse, as it seems more likely—was just decimated by my friend's pregnancy. Hers was the first but not the only one. It felt like almost weekly that another mom in our gymnastics or swimming class announced she was expecting. I could no longer claim it was too soon; my peers proved that was untrue.

The question nagged at me. Left me with a feeling of unease. I was happy for them, but at the same time I was jealous. Plain and simple, I didn't need my therapist or months of reflection to decipher the underlying cause of my emotions. While I wasn't ready to admit it out loud, I knew in my heart that I wanted another baby. At least I wanted to try.

I buried my desire—same as I had been doing for months. Only now I *knew* I'd been burying it. I was afraid of saying anything. What if my husband didn't agree with me? Would hearing him say no be harder than not knowing?

We carried on with our dance of denial. Every so often one of us would broach the subject and just as quickly dismiss it as a joke. Sort of like "Hey, I think I'm ovulating. Who wants to put a baby in me?" Pause. "I'm kidding! Of course." Or my husband would come to bed at night, put his arm around me and ask, "Shall we try to give Archer a baby brother or sister?" Before my eyes could register a look of confusion, wondering whether this was real or a joke, he'd follow his words with the same disclaimer I always used: "Just kidding!"

I can't remember who first broke the spell, but if forced to guess, I'd say it was my husband. He has a great knack for delicately broaching awkward topics, whereas I'm the stereotypical bull in a china shop. I vaguely recall his approaching the topic as we always had before, only he left off the "just kidding" ending. The conversation was back on the table.

We admitted to one another that we wanted another child but didn't know if we should. Yes, our age was a concern, but the real reason we were hesitating was the PPD. It was hard to forget the fact that for a period of time I'd wanted to take my own life. We didn't ignore it; we couldn't. We had to face it head-on—once again—and factor that into our decision.

Though it's easy to forget just *how* bad things have been. My mother always told me I'd romanticize even the worst relationships after a breakup.

I tend to gloss over the bad parts and carry forward with only the good. A glaring problem. I need to remember; it's how I'll grow and move forward. This case was no exception.

I bought a journal and began writing down everything from that dark period just after Archer had been born. The hateful thoughts. How I'd felt toward my son. My husband. Myself. All the pain I could recall having felt. As I sat down to read through my notes, I was expecting the worst. I thought it would break my heart, send me down a spiral and make me not want to try again.

It didn't. Yes, it made me sad. My heart broke for her, the woman who had suffered so much. But I was no longer that person. Now I knew more; I'd put together quite the robust tool kit to work on my PPD since the day my son had been born. One I still carry with me everywhere I go, and I know when I need to use it.

Looking back, I can see now that I had gone into battle unarmed. And it *was* a battle; I had been fighting against PPD for my life. I had known nothing of the enemy or how to take it down. Each time it attacked me, I had been vulnerable and unexposed. At first, that is. On the day I went to ask my doctor for help, I stopped fighting alone. And by the time my son's first birthday came around, I was a true warrior. I had my shield up, my weapons ready, and I knocked down each setback. And it was easier and easier each time.

I wondered, would I be better equipped to face PPD the second time around? If it even were to happen again. That's the thing, of course—there's a chance it would return. Statistics say it probably could. Oh, but what if it didn't? What if I were one of those unicorn women, the ones who stay healthy and happy postpartum? Who are present and able to enjoy their newborn child?

It might not happen that way. But it could. Instead of staying in the "never again" lane, my husband and I slowly merged into "maybe."

We spoke with my doctor and therapist. I reached out to other women I'd become close to with who also endured PPD. I exhausted every resource, listened to countless stories, and weighed endless opinions. At the end of the day, however, the final decision was still ours.

I always wait for the other shoe to drop. I try to be positive, but I do start to think it's inevitable. Which is probably why, as things were progressing so positively, I was overcome with guilt. I felt like I was being selfish to everyone around me. I was planning to walk into a fire and expect others to be there to help me if I were burned.

I mentioned this to my husband, and he paused before he spoke. It wasn't a good sign. "I've been thinking the same thing," he confessed. "Maybe we *shouldn't* try for a second one. I'm not sure anymore, either."

I was heartbroken. He was the one who was supposed to be sure. I needed him strong and decisive so *I* could waffle. One of us had to be decisive; there wasn't room for both of us to be unsure. I wanted to have hold of the long rope that would allow me to go back and forth on our decision, but he wasn't supposed to waver. No, he was supposed to be sure. I was still afraid to say that I wanted this, because I felt guilty over what we'd all gone through the first time.

But now, with my husband's indecision, somehow the answer emerged right in front of me: yes, with a side of guilt. It was only in hindsight—now that my husband was taking the option off the table—that I could see what I really wanted. I had been putting all the blame on myself and deciding I wasn't allowed to want—or maybe wasn't worthy of wanting—a second child. Which is why I had been secretly hoping my husband would want to try again. He had a right to want—I didn't. In a way, I had been seeking his approval on the plan before I felt like I could cosign. And I hadn't understood this in time.

And so no became our answer. But all the while my heart was screaming otherwise. I couldn't silence the part of me that wanted another child. Children aren't an accessory, and we're not entitled to have as many as we'd like. I know I need to think of my family, I'd tell myself. But then I'd watch my son cradle his baby dolls, feeding and kissing them. He'd begun asking for a baby sister. In my heart I knew I wasn't done.

I needed to find a way to reconcile my desire to have a second child with the guilt of the potential burden I might be placing upon my family. My anxiety usually takes over in moments like this; I tend to assume the worst and decide by indecision. "I haven't decided yet," I'll tell myself. But who am I kidding? That's the cowardly way out. After enough time, *not deciding* is your answer.

My forty-third birthday was then upon us, and it was hard to pretend we didn't know what that meant. *Ticktock* went the sound of my fertility. It was now or never, so I simply asked my husband what he wanted to do.

"I want to have another baby, but I thought you were done." His answer felt like a question.

Ping. The ball was in my court.

"I want another child. I want Archer to have a sibling," I said, finally dropping the ifs and buts from my answers and being honest.

Pong. The ball went back to him.

I expected him to defer, give me one of our signature "I'm just kidding" follow-ups. Instead, he looked at me stoically and asked what steps I thought we should take. It was the beginning of a conversation that was certainly long but perhaps not as hard as I'd expected. We discussed our options, whether we should explore fertility assistance, and the timing, even reflecting on how trying to conceive the first time had made our sex life feel like a job.

It was an honest and cathartic talk for both of us. But there were still two more people I needed to talk with: my parents.

I'm a big believer in community. I can't and won't try to raise my son without help. Whether it's family or just another mom friend stepping in to watch him while I run out to get my eyebrows waxed (because self-care is important!), we can't do it alone. We knew that even if I were able to keep any future PPD at bay, we'd need help.

My parents had been the compass for our journey; we wouldn't have made it to the other side without them. They had stayed with us so my husband could go to work and I wouldn't be alone, driven ten hours in one day to pick up me and my son when my husband had had to go on a business trip, given everything they could to help us. I'd be remiss if I thought I could do it again without them. The question was, were they ready?

It wasn't fair of me to assume they'd be willing (and able) to support us through a potential second round of PPD. I needed to discuss it with them, to hear their thoughts. If they didn't think they could be as involved again, we'd need to factor that into our decision.

I poured my heart out to them. My fears and desires, my concern that I wouldn't be able to do it without them if it happened again. I must have been a good person in a previous life to deserve them, because they said yes without hesitation. "Yes, 100 percent," to be specific.

At last I had all my weapons. My army was assembled and standing behind me. I knew I was ready to face whatever might come, and that same night I stopped taking my birth control.

That was in the late summer of 2018, just one month before Archer's second birthday.

My grandmother passed away several years ago at a hundred years old, when I was about four months pregnant with Archer. Her motto had been "What's meant to be is meant to be." In the spirit of her words, now we shall see what we will as we continue to try for baby number two. Officially.

HANNAH, TWENTY-SIX YEARS OLD

It was the early morning of December 15, 2015, and I had been laboring for almost ten hours. I was shaky, depleted, exhausted, but so determined. I had walked through the slow and calm contractions of early labor and then wrestled with the intensity of active labor for hours. I thought—I hoped—that I was close to the end. At around 9, my midwife asked me to get onto my back so that she could check my cervix. Even though I really didn't want to, I complied. With the help of my birthing team, I hoisted myself up from a sumo-squat position and laid my weak body back onto a stack of pillows.

After some movement and *a lot* of discomfort, she uttered the words, "I have some bad news."

"Shit," I thought to myself.

"You're only three centimeters," confirming my fears.

Shit. I had never known such defeat. Up until this moment, the contractions had been rushing in, one on top of the other. Like waves they would sweep in, tackle me to the ground and leave me more drained than before. Then, before I could stand up, another would come in and knock me right back on my ass. But it seemed that after this news, it all stopped for a moment. I computed what the midwife had told me while my emotions arrived and decided they'd take over. The tears started pouring out as if the dam within me had broken, and they just kept coming.

For the first time since I had begun laboring, I lost my composure completely and let myself really *feel*. I wanted to quit. I wanted to make the contractions stop. I wanted to be done.

But the not-so-funny thing about laboring is that there is only one way out when you're already in it. You can't go over it, you can't go around it, you have to go through it.

I knew I had no choice but to pull my shit together and go back to work. My mom-doubled-doula told me it was time to battle again and push through, just as a contraction started to rear its ugly head. Several hours and another cervix check later, I was ten centimeters dilated and knew it was finally time to finish the climb once and for all. My midwife had just broken my water, and the pushing train was pulling in to the station quickly. I was so desperately ready to make the pain end. But pushing meant that soon I'd be giving birth. Giving birth meant actually seeing my baby. I was going to meet my son. I was going to be *a mom*. Was I even ready for that?

Of course, this story had begun months earlier, in my boyfriend's bathroom, as I'd stared at two *very* solid lines. I remember the rush of shock and fear that had hit me instantaneously and how the world had suddenly felt as if it were closing in around me. My vision had become tunneled, and my heart had raced.

"There's no way this is real. There's no way this is happening to me. I'm trapped, and there's no way out of this. No matter what I do from this moment on, I will be forever changed," I'd thought. My partner, DJ, was standing there with me, but there was no dialogue between us. Just silence. My mind was going crazy, as I'm sure his was, but we didn't utter any words of fear to each other. The way I remember it, we'd sat in silence for what felt like a lifetime. We were stunned and terrified but both immediately knew our lives would never be the same.

DJ and I had broken up two weeks prior to finding out we were pregnant. We had been dating for about six months, and the relationship hadn't been working functionally for most of that time. We were alike and compatible in so many ways, but so very opposite in others. We stood on opposite sides of the fence a lot of the time, and neither of us was really willing to budge on our differences. We were two young people so desperately in love but so very different. As heartbroken as we'd been, we had tired of fighting and knew we would need to cut our losses and move forward. Or so we'd thought.

From the moment of that pregnancy test until about twelve weeks into the pregnancy, life consisted of utter turmoil and indecision. DJ pushed for me to terminate the pregnancy, stemming from his feelings of fear and uncertainty. Some days I was right there with him. Other days I was half-heartedly "ready" to move forward with the pregnancy and have a baby. I felt helpless and trapped. All paths seemed like they would contain complete loss and devastation. I sat with my family, his family, and my therapist for weeks, trying to figure out the right answer. Adoption, abortion, or raising a child. I weighed each option so heavily, trying each one on and playing out the ending in my head. The future felt grim no matter which ending I envisioned.

After weeks of wrestling with this new reality, my therapist brought me to my answer with two simple questions.

She asked, "What scares you most about having a baby?"

To which I answered, "I'm scared of how hard it will be, but I know that I can do it, and in the end, I know with certainty I'll be okay."

She then asked, "What is your biggest fear about terminating the pregnancy?"

And I answered, "I'm afraid if I go through with it, I'll never be okay again." She didn't even have to respond for me to realize that I had just found my answer.

The next several months were nothing short of a total shit show. It took months of freaking out before DJ was able to come around and actually join me in the pregnancy and planning for the future. Those few months were some of the hardest of my life. I not only felt completely alone and terrified, but the one person I so needed and wanted to have by my side wanted nothing to do with me or this baby. I was angry with him—hated him, almost—but only because I needed him and the comfort only he could offer me. I look back and feel bad that I couldn't understand his fight-or-flight reaction. He was a single, twenty-five-year-old guy who was just about to graduate college. He didn't have a "grown-up" job. He didn't have his life figured out. And he had always planned to not marry or settle down until he was at least thirty. Of course he was freaked out.

As for me, I began the pregnancy scared and ashamed. I didn't want to tell anyone, out of fear that they would judge and condemn me for my lack of responsibility. I was ashamed that I had gotten pregnant unplanned, which left me feeling disgusted with myself and the baby I was growing. As my body changed and the world started to slowly find out, I still remained resentful of this growing life inside of me. It took months for me to adjust to the idea of being pregnant and becoming a mom—months of paralyzing fear, uncertainty, and shame. But eventually that all changed. Over time I grew fonder of my growing belly. My friends encouraged me to take photos of my pregnant body, and I didn't squirm. My family was celebrating me and showering me with love and support, and I actually started to join them. I was no longer heartbroken. I was actually becoming *excited*. It had taken so much time, but I was getting there.

DJ came around too, and we were able to plan and prepare together for what was left of the pregnancy.

In that time, I moved out of my house where I had been living with three of my best girlfriends and in with my mom. I then moved out of my mom's house and in with DJ in his parents' house. We then moved out of their house and into our own condo a mere three days before our due date. The stress of all of that moving and uncertainty took a real toll on my health and mental state. When the "nesting period" of my pregnancy came, I couldn't nest because I didn't know where my nest was going to be. I washed and folded all of the clothes we'd gotten for the baby but had nowhere to put them away. I bought and handmade decorations for a nursery but didn't have a space to decorate. I wanted so desperately to settle in somewhere, like all moms do (I thought), but I couldn't.

I know with great confidence that it was *all* of the stress of my pregnancy, from the indecision and shame to the uncertainty of our living situation, that led me to the dark place I ended up after having our son.

In the end, on that day in the hospital, I pushed for only forty-five minutes before my sweet little boy's head was earth-side, his body ready to follow. As an aside, the ring of fire that they teach you about in birthing classes is a *very* real thing. There was a moment in between his head being birthed and the rest of his body—a moment of pause. I was able to feel him moving around inside and outside of me at the same time. It was simultaneously the most beautiful and the weirdest feeling I'd ever felt. With one more deep breath, I pushed him out and brought him up onto my chest.

The moments following were the most euphoric and profound of my whole entire life. The instant relief and rush of emotions were completely overwhelming but in the best way possible. I had climbed the most insurmountable mountain and come out with the best gift of all—new life. There is nothing on this earth that can prepare you for what that feels like, and there is absolutely nothing that compares. On December 15, at 3:29 P.M., we met our Oliver David, and he was beautiful.

I laid with my baby boy on my chest for hours upon hours, and everything else seemed to melt away. It was just the two of us in our bubble, soaking each other in. It was different from how I'd always imagined it, though. Most people had led me to believe that this euphoria would last forever and that I would be in love with this new, little being instantly.

But it didn't, and I wasn't.

The love I felt for this little baby was all-encompassing and huge but so unfamiliar. As much as I loved him completely by nature, I didn't know him at all. He was beautiful, but if I'm being honest, I wasn't in love. The truth is, we were strangers, and I felt that so deeply. It felt scary to feel differently from how I'd thought I was *supposed* to feel.

Was I a bad mom already?

Was I unfit?

Would I ever connect with him the way I was expected to?

Hours went by, and my thoughts kept racing. But now, instead of just being concerned about our lack of connection, my thoughts were also racing elsewhere. Instead of just being consumed by one thing, I was growing petrified of a million others. My hand remained planted on his chest or back at all times, in fear that he was going to stop breathing. I had a running stream of thoughts in my head of all the ways he could die. In an instant, my existence was so dependent on this human that I didn't even know, and the enormity of that scared the hell out of me. Quickly, the paranoia about his death turned into fear of my own death and DJ's death. I laid awake for days and nights with this fear and panic within me, knowing it was completely irrational but unable to control it at all. When I say I was awake for days and nights, I mean it literally.

Everyone told me, "Nap when the baby naps," and I wanted to, but I couldn't. My mind would not let me rest. I thought that if I went to sleep, I surely would not wake up. I thought that if I went to sleep, I would miss him somehow dying when I could have otherwise saved him. This paranoia and fear left me sleep deprived and pushed me further into a state of utter delusion.

After a few days of horrible suffering internally, I let my mom and DJ in on my fears and thoughts. They encouraged and led me to share them with my midwife, who was still coming over almost daily for postpartum checkups. I opened up to her, and she explained that a lot of what I was feeling could still fall under the blanket term "baby blues." From what I understand and was told, the baby-blues period was from birth until about three weeks postpartum. Apparently if you are still in that time frame, your symptoms are not really taken seriously as anything more than a normal hormonal shift. She said that my symptoms should subside and that if they didn't by four weeks, they would assess me further. She gave me some natural tinctures to help keep the anxiety at bay, but as I'm sure you can already assume, they did not work.

The next few weeks came and went, and instead of improving, my symptoms only got worse. I had spiraled into a state of complete paranoia and panic and had almost lost touch with reality entirely. I was feeling anxious, paranoid, and incapacitated with fear in addition to feeling an unfamiliar feeling I now know as derealization: I felt completely out of my body, almost as if I were floating and watching from above. My vision was distorted, and so was my hearing. I couldn't hold a conversation, as I would immediately lose track and forget the sentence I or the other person was saying as it left their mouths.

As things progressed, I began to hear voices in my head. They started as a dull mumbling, almost as if there were multiple people whispering inside my head all at once. I vividly remember sitting in the rocking chair, nursing Ollie, trying to make out what the voices were telling me. There were messages being conveyed, but I couldn't translate them. All of this left me completely beside myself. But instead of telling everyone *all* that I had been experiencing, I hid it, only sharing the bare minimum. I'm the kind of person who likes to keep my composure. I like to be in control, and I like to be "strong." I hated feeling so out of control and didn't want anyone to really know how deeply I was suffering. I thought that if I only told them I was experiencing panic and anxiety along with some depression, I'd be given medication and would go back to my normal self quickly, without anyone having to know how lost I really was. I have never been so wrong in my life, and that is what led to me suffering for the better half of my son's first year.

One night, in the midst of all this mess, as we came home from a dinner out, I started to feel something unlike anything I had felt before. The world started to spin and shift on its axis, and my vision became quickly blurred. The voices that I had been hearing in my head went from a dull mumble to an unbearable roar, and I couldn't hear anything but the noise that filled my head. I felt as though I were in the midst of a horrible storm, as if I were sitting in the eye of a tornado, hanging on to only a small piece of debris. I tried to tell DJ what was going on but couldn't stabilize or get grounded enough to communicate.

At that same exact moment, Ollie started screaming incessantly. I've always felt that he and I were connected on a level deeper than I could fully comprehend. When I was suffering most, he was also distressed. When I was calm, he was at ease. So it was no surprise that he began screaming and crying in my very worst moments. He needed me to soothe him the way only I, as his mother, could. I tried desperately to nurse and pacify him, but I just could not. I pushed him away, back into DJ's arms, and ran to the bathroom to try and escape this hell. I sat on the toilet, trying to find my bearings, and that's when I saw him: Jesus, standing in my bathroom, looking back at me.

That episode landed me in front of a psychiatrist the very next day, and I was evaluated for one hour. I poured my heart and symptoms out to her, chronicling everything from the moment I gave birth to my son to the moment of "the episode." After word-vomiting for an hour, it took her all of one moment to give me a clear and concise answer.

"You have postpartum psychosis," she said with utter certainty.

And from then on, I began my healing journey.

The healing process, for me, began with that diagnosis. I had wasted so much time misleading my doctors, which had led them to an initial inadequate diagnosis—and, even worse, a period of time with no diagnosis at all. But now I was on the right path—the path to wellness. The medications prescribed to me by the psychiatrist, although many, were all to treat the correct illness. Instead of going on more SSRIs to treat depression and anxiety—which, as listed as a potential side effect, can ironically push you further into psychosis—I was put on antipsychotics and mood stabilizers. Inch by inch, I was recovering. I spent the next eight months easing onto medications and then weaning off, only to ease onto new ones. You see, medications to treat mental illness are anything but one-size-fits-all. It's all about finding the right fit, and for me that took months. Eventually I was put on a mood stabilizer called Lamictal and on an antipsychotic called Abilify, and things began to click. I had found my groove, and I was slowly finding a new and healthy "normal." It was gradual, and anything but linear, but I healed. Boy, did I heal.

My life post-postpartum psychosis continued to be messy but also so, so beautiful. My relationship with Ollie's dad, DJ, ended again, but this time for good. It was a hard but also a sweet and mature parting, followed by a rocky journey to establishing a healthy co-parenting relationship. I lost my nuclear family and in turn found my independence, which, if I'm being honest, I had never really known before. The transformation I went through was brutal but so necessary and so gratifying.

Following my separation, I reconnected with the sweetest man I had (have) ever known, Christopher. The connection between us had been instant, but the timing wasn't right for us to come together. We spent a few months on a pretty fierce roller coaster, with my indecision and confusion leading the way. I was hot and then cold, yes and then no. I was a real-life Katy Perry song. And yet he hung on. He stayed, and he was there through the poor timing and all that came with it. He was there by my side while I mourned the loss of the family I had so dreamed of having and was so gracious and understanding, regardless of what that meant for him. He knew that he wasn't going to be my first priority, and he supported that. He knew that I came with baggage and would always be a package deal, and he embraced that. He loved that Ollie came first for me and respected the fact that DJ was an integral piece to my puzzle. He held space for DJ as my co-parent and Ollie's dad. He never imposed his thoughts or feelings about our situation or my parenting, and he was careful to never step on anyone's toes. He handled a heavy circumstance with such grace and dignity, and I will never forget how that made me feel.

But most important, of course, was the way he loved my son. Their connection was natural and easy from the start. It was never forced or pushed. It was always genuine and real. Christopher stepped into Ollie's life as a bonus figure who cared for him, nurtured him, taught him, and truly, deeply loved him. I grew from mourning the loss of the family unit we'd once been to feeling thankful for all the changes that had led us to our Christopher. He was meant for us and we for him. For all those reasons and then some, I knew he was someone I needed to hold onto. What had started as a true and deep friendship turned into a beautiful and new family.

In our first months together, Christopher and I fell deeper in love, nourished our new family bond, traveled, changed jobs, established new friendships, and held each other close. We experienced the joy and gratification of buying a home and planting our roots together, and we continued to plan our beautiful future together. Talk of marriage emerged, and just as newer couples do, we quickly got down to business dreaming up the rest of our life. First comes love, then comes marriage, then comes . . . well, you know. When we approached the topic of growing our family, I froze.

I had always dreamed of having multiple children. I'd wanted at least three, but maybe more. A boy, a girl, two of each—or anything, really. *That* was my dream. I had always had expectations and fantasies about motherhood and what that would look like for me. I had watched friends and family members close to me have babies, and I'd seen the bliss and happiness they felt afterward. I'd watched them breastfeed with ease, endure sleepless nights with grace, and triumph with their child at each milestone they reached. When my time had come, I'd expected all of that but instead had felt anguish and misery. Breastfeeding had been stressful and difficult, and of course I hadn't had the capacity to deal with it gracefully. We had pushed through that and triumphed over the hurdles because it was so important to me. But with every change of medication, our breastfeeding relationship was called into question anew, and my heart would break. Through Ollie's milestone achievements I had been fighting for my life. I hadn't been able to enjoy them the way I'd always dreamed, and now either I cannot remember them or their memory brings me feelings of disgust and makes me sick to my stomach.

My experience of being a new mommy had been nothing short of a living hell, and I swore I would never, ever do it again. All of the dreaming and fantasizing I had done my whole life had all been burned to the ground. Here I was, with my one beautiful child, swearing that I would never have another. But now that Chris was in my life and future, I was no longer certain. I felt pressure to have the answer right away, assuming he needed that. I wanted so badly to be able to "provide" him with the option of growing our family, and I felt like I would be disappointing him if I couldn't. We talked and talked and then talked some more. He stressed relentlessly that no matter what, he would be completely content with our family. He assured me time and time again that our family was more than enough for him right where we stood. He told me that Ollie was *his* son now too, fulfilling any dreams he'd of having children of his own. More than anything, he stressed that he would never want me to experience the darkness that I'd lived for the sake of doing what I thought he wanted. But I did not—could not—accept his answer. I had convinced myself long before these conversations that he would need us to have a child together, and so it didn't really matter how much he tried to sway me in the other direction. Having set my heart on that truth, I couldn't hear, or didn't listen to, what he was saying.

We spent so much time discussing this huge and overwhelming topic, per my pushing, until he finally got through to me. I finally understood that his desire, truly, was to maintain my health and happiness and that nothing else mattered more. Ultimately, we both decided that this would be an ever-growing and -changing decision and that, since we weren't "at that bridge yet," we could wait to face it when it really came time.

Two years have come and gone. Two years of growth, change, love, and, still, indecision. As Ollie has grown older, people have been constantly asking The Questions:

"Are you going to have more babies?"

"Don't you want Ollie to have a sibling?"

"Does Chris want to have a baby of his own?"

You name it, I've heard it. And the truth still remains: I have *no idea* what any of the answers are. I have been in a place of such turmoil and limbo that my answer really depends on which day you ask me or what side of the bed I woke up on. Some days I've had such fierce baby fever that I could have gotten pregnant just by looking at Chris. Other days I've had panic attacks at just the thought of it. Months at a time pass and I will be utterly convinced that I had picked our path, and then, like the flip of a switch, it will change again. The inner conflict consumes me. But more present and powerful than all of the fear is my longing to have another baby of my own. Selfishly, maybe, I want a second chance. I want my shot at a redemption song. I wanted to *try* and *plan* to get pregnant, and I wanted to be over-the-moon excited when I see those two very solid lines. I want to feel proud and eager to tell our families and anticipate their joy. I want to embrace and love when my body grows and changes. I want to cry with overwhelming happiness when I feel a baby kick for the first time, and I want to experience a partner who is there with me to feel it. I want to take pregnancy photos. I want to beam openly with pride at the baby we've created. I want to give Chris a baby that is ours, together. I want to give Ollie the irreplaceable bond of a sibling. I want to give birth confidently, knowing that I am ready to be a mother, because I already am a damn good one. I want to feel peace and calm seeing my baby's face for the first time. I want to lay in postbirth bliss for what feels like an eternity, as the world passes me by without my even knowing. I want to fall in love all over again, no matter how long it takes, without the disturbance of loud voices in my head. I want serenity. I want peace. I want the experience that I have earned and feel like I deserve.

Being the numbers-based person that I am, I did my research. One in one thousand. That is the chance of a woman getting postpartum psychosis. I was that one. The odds were almost completely in my favor, and I still got dealt this hand. So, in considering growing our family, I also have to consider the likelihood that my psychosis would repeat itself the second time around. One in two. Fifty percent of women who've had postpartum psychosis previously will have another "episode" after their next pregnancy. After considering this all to myself, and then discussing it with Chris for a while, I took these statistics to my doctor, hoping to come find some more concrete answers than the ones Google had given me. We sat in her office, and she told me, frankly, that I would probably deal with a reoccurrence of psychosis. But she was also able to give me a wealth of information that helped me feel more optimistic and hopeful. She reassured me about that which I already knew: *Having experienced postpartum psychosis previously, you are far more equipped to deal with it. You know the signs and symptoms and will be able to notice them and name them from the second they begin. There are preventative measures, such as getting on medications late in your pregnancy to hopefully prevent or at least manage it before it begins. And of course, once you've given birth, there are even more options of treatment that are safe during breastfeeding.* I can't explain the contrast of relief and dread that I felt leaving her office that day. Those emotions carried me out her door and through my everyday life for months. I had more information but, still, so much to consider.

It has officially been three and a half years since I began my journey with postpartum mental illness. I have spent the better portion of that time wrestling with the idea, day in and day out, of growing our family. I am faced with multiple paths that all feel like they would end in happiness and contentment but that also paralyze me with fear. After battling and sitting with this inner conflict for so long, I think I've finally reached a point of clarity. The answer to the question of whether to grow our family is that there is no answer. Unsatisfying? Yes. Uncertain? Certainly. Open ended? Very much so. But somehow I have found comfort in the unknown. I understand that the ending for my book has not yet been written. I am okay with the fact that today's feelings could be the polar opposite of tomorrow's. For now I will continue to do my mental puzzle. I will continue to long for a baby. I will continue to fear it as well. I will continue to feel all the things I need to feel, and I will trust that it will all happen the way it should, and that, no matter what, we will all be happy and successful. If I am to choose to bear more children, and should I suffer again, I will persevere just the way I did after my first baby.

And, again, I will come out stronger, wiser, and more capable than before. If I choose not to grow our family, I will triumph through that with grace and power, knowing with confidence that we were only meant to be a family of three. I certainly don't know the ending to my family's story, but what I do know is that with it will come unwavering strength, unconditional love, and impenetrable peace. And that is more than any mother could ever want—much more. I have a dream future husband who loves me and my son unconditionally, and I have a beautiful son who is beyond what I could have ever imagined for myself and more. Most important, I have the family unit I have always dreamed of and longed for, and no matter where this life takes us, with more babies or not, we will all feel complete. And that is my beautiful truth.

SAMANTHA, THIRTY-THREE YEARS OLD

I was exactly thirty-eight weeks pregnant and at a routine checkup when my blood-pressure reading came back uncharacteristically high. I was in for a general, weekly, end-of-pregnancy checkup, but when the doctors saw my readings, they rushed me to the hospital to be admitted. They decided that it was best for me to have my labor induced, as the baby was full-term. It felt like what must have been one of the longest inductions in the twenty-first century. I'm not sure if that's actually fact, but I can't imagine it any other way. My labor induction began on a Monday morning, and I didn't end up delivering the baby until Wednesday. A seventy-two-hour labor was not what I'd had in mind as a birth plan. After the doctors did everything they could to speed up my dilatation process—both with manual manipulations in the beginning and then later with a medicine used to increase the frequency and force of contractions—it was clear that the dilation was not working for me.

After this long labor, in every sense of the word, my medical team suggested an emergency C-section, informing me that the baby's heart rate was beginning to be of concern. At that point, I was thrilled to just get cut open. I remember the extreme, excruciating pain of those hours of back labor as equal only to the extreme, excruciatingly terrible thoughts I began to have about myself and the baby.

I asked myself and my husband a seemingly endless stream of questions. Most important, I can remember asking, on repeat, "Are the baby and I going to be okay?"

I can so vividly recall the sound of the countless other mothers' babies' first cries, as all around us, in the labor-and-delivery unit, they were being born, while we were just stuck waiting. These cries continued from Monday evening until I was prepped for my C-section surgery Wednesday. I just kept thinking how ready and excited I was to finally meet my baby.

As I waited for the moment of truth, the doctors reentered the room, which I assumed was to wheel me out to the operating room. But to my surprise, they explained that the C-section was off the table. I was finally dilating, and quickly, and so I was going to have to push my baby out. My husband and I were so confused, but we just continued to field the constant curveballs and roll with the punches, so to speak. Within the next few hours, I dilated fully and was ready to push.

This was the most painful part of it all. From the moment I'd found out I was pregnant, I'd planned to get an epidural. But, like everything else, not even my pain management went as planned. By the time I was told to start pushing, alongside a team of six doctors, I was under so much stress that my body and mind were not working together. The combination of adrenaline and exhaustion had hurled me into fight-or-flight mode. My body decided to fight to get her out of me; however, my mind wasn't working fast enough. Because of my burgeoning anxiety, I completely forgot to ask for more epidural medicine. I was so focused on getting my baby out of me alive and surviving this delivery that I was incapable of meeting my body's most basic needs.

And, yes, I felt everything. And, yes, it was the most pain I have ever endured.

But beyond the physical pain was the emotional pain. The worry. After two hours of aggressive pushing, my daughter was born. I remember my first feeling of a maternal instinct kicking in, and I immediately wanted to have her right there next to me. I held her and looked into her face, still unable to believe all that had happened and all that was to come. But my daughter didn't cry. My whole life, I had thought that a healthy baby lets out a big cry right after being born. When this did not happen, I started to feel panicky. Finally, after what seemed like an eternity, but was probably not even a minute, the cry came.

When my daughter was whisked away from me, taken by the nurses for evaluation and such, I swung to the opposite end of the emotional spectrum, and instead of wanting her as close to me as possible, I was overwhelmed by the sense of relief when she was taken away. I had always imagined that the moment after I had a baby I would want her right next to me. I would want to breastfeed her. I would want to kiss her. But in reality, I wanted for her to be taken away. And for that I felt extremely guilty. I chalked this feeling up to my nightmarish delivery and prepared myself for what I thought was to come.

The strangest thing I remember is that right after delivery, while I was holding my new baby girl in my arms, my doctor looked me right in the eyes and told me that I would have postpartum depression.

Yes, that's right. Without even knowing my past mental-health history, the doctors predicted I would get postpartum depression based upon my delivery alone. Little did we know.

After April 26, 2017, when I delivered my beautiful, perfectly healthy baby girl, an internal switch flipped in my brain. She was all I had wanted, and then suddenly I wanted nothing to do with her. There was no initial connection or euphoria. Just looking at her, let alone holding her, gave me stress, uncertainty, and an overall depressive feeling.

It didn't help that I was attached to a catheter for the first few days after the delivery and therefore stuck in the hospital bed, making it so that I could not stand up to change diapers or walk around or do any basic tasks. My body was so swollen from the preeclampsia (the cause of my high blood pressure) that I could barely walk, even if I'd been allowed. I remember looking down at my legs and feet and seeing that they were so swollen that they literally looked like big balloons. They were so misshapen that it was hard even for my parents to look at my legs and feet, which only served to further my feelings of isolation. Though I desperately wanted to physically be deflated from my massive water retention, the doctors told me it would take weeks for this to happen. Another blow.

After the delivery, I felt like I had survived a war. Truthfully, I was still concerned with myself and whether I was going to be okay both mentally and physically. The doctors at the hospital kept pushing breastfeeding on me. Forget about breastfeeding—I could barely be joyful that I'd just had a baby! It was like a cruel joke. I couldn't even get out of the hospital bed to change a diaper, and yet they wanted me to learn how to breastfeed. I remember staring back at them like they were speaking a foreign language as they suggested breastfeeding positions and offered lactation advice. I kept trying to put my daughter to my boob, but I wasn't producing milk, and so my insecurity only grew. The thing that was supposed to be natural felt like the least instinctual process for my baby and for me.

Once I was finally allowed to be discharged, I remember dressing my daughter in her "take-home outfit" at the hospital but being scared shitless at the thought of actually taking this baby home. I immediately felt so much pressure and anxiety—self-doubt. I believed that I would mess up being a mom. When we returned home and visitors came to see my beautiful bundle, I so desperately tried to play the part and adjust to this, my role as a mom.

I could not.

I could not bond with her, despite my best efforts. It was so bad that I could barely hold her, or even go near her, without crying or second-guessing my parenting skills.

"Having a baby was the worst mistake I have ever made," I thought to myself, with a combination of resolve and shame.

This made me feel like a monster and set off the worst part of my story. I was so depressed, and burdened by such guilt, that I became suicidal. I did not want to get out of bed, as life seemed too trying and painful. As a matter of survival, my husband and I, together, decided to go against the doctors' urging, and I quit trying to breastfeed so that I could begin taking medication. This was an emergency. We knew that my daughter could be fed with formula, and it was much more important to try to get me healthier.

During those first few months of her life, I cannot begin to express the guilt that plagued me.

"Why do I feel this way?"

"This definitely, without a doubt, means I am the worst mother and don't even deserve a chance to be her mom."

"I don't deserve to wake up each day to this family."

These thoughts would circle in my mind constantly. I would not wish the pain I felt during the first four months of my daughter's life on anyone.

It was pure hell and misery. I felt so stuck in my thoughts and mind, and I also felt like nothing was helping. I went from one doctor to another, and then I went to one treatment center to the next, but nothing seemed to ease my pain.

I was going in circles. I had no release, I had no treatments that were working correctly, and I was so confused about how something I had dreamed about my entire life could be so opposite to what I had expected. Why had I dreamed of being a mom since I was a little girl if being a mom was like *this*?

I could not get out of bed. I was not a functioning human. Deep in my postpartum depression, my enjoyment for everything I had enjoyed before my baby had disappeared. I had lost myself. I had lost the desire to live. My siblings, parents, husband, and those closest to me felt as if I had disappeared. I no longer cared about spending time with my husband, my dog, my family, or my new baby. Before motherhood, I had been a positive, goofy, happy-go-lucky person, and it was as if I had forgotten how to smile.

With my depression I could not pay attention enough to or read or watch TV, so I had no distraction from my thoughts. I stopped talking to anyone. I did not go outside. Knowing that my situation was dire, I begged my mom and husband to take me to a mental hospital. They told me to be patient and that things would get better and to just "hang in there."

They told me *no*.

Without their support for a higher level of care, I had no hope that things would ever get better, and so I convinced myself that life would be better without me. These were my darkest days. I felt as if I were on a ship sinking further and further into a storm with no way out. I could not look at myself in the mirror during these times, and I lost all hope that things would get better. All of the medications that the psychiatrists placed me on were doing nothing to ease my feelings of despair. I now know that I was suffering from severe postpartum OCD (obsessive-compulsive disorder) and severe postpartum depression.

Thankfully, one family member—my cousin—stepped in and advocated for my hospitalization. Amid the agony I was experiencing, I was so thankful that at least one person was listening, and for this I will be forever grateful. I was admitted to emergency hospitalization for three weeks. It was essential for me to be in a hospital, as I needed to be monitored closely, both physically and mentally, during this time. The hospital also gave me a completely new team of doctors to weigh in on my situation and recommend new medicine. These doctors consistently reassured me that I would be okay and would come out of my suffering once the right medication was in my system.

I can remember being all alone in my hospital room with pictures of my daughter, my husband, and my dog surrounding me and crying so hard that I was shaking.

"Am I ever going to pull through this?" I wondered.

"Am I going to be okay?"

During this time I knew that my daughter was being cared for by my mother, and so I knew she was in wonderful hands. I would call as much as I could to get updates as to how she was doing, so now, looking back on it, I realize how much I cared about her but that it was manifesting in the form of fear. I felt so scared for myself, along with tremendous guilt and anxiety. Though this was my rock bottom, my lowest of lows, I truly believe that I needed to get to that point in my story to begin to rise above it.

After the being released from the hospital after my weeks-long stay, I started a treatment of full-time cognitive behavioral therapy. Between the clinical help and the medicine, I slowly started to believe that I would get better with time, and I started consciously fighting my mental illness. I believe that the right medicine that they gave me kicked in, which helped tremendously to ease up my symptoms. Slowly I became myself again. Day by day, with a lot of support, a lot of treatment, and a lot of hard work, I came back to life. I started taking care of my daughter with the help of others, and I started to get more comfortable with accepting the fact that I needed help for her. That it was okay for me to go to therapy and to work out while someone else was taking care of her. That this didn't make me a bad mom at all. I learned that making good decisions for myself and providing self-care for myself were best for her well-being as well as my own.

As a mom I worked on bonding with my daughter, making decisions for her, and making her needs a priority. I started to have more confidence with my decisions and used positive self-talk to get me through those uncomfortable and stressful parenting moments. I learned how to ground myself and use my senses as ways to stay present instead of being caught up in the junk that spins through my head. I made a promise to myself and those closest to me that I would continue to work hard to beat my OCD.

One thing that I want everyone to know is that that the deep love for my daughter was always there in my heart. I have always loved her to the moon and back. During my suffering, I just genuinely thought that her life would be better without me in it. I now know that this is not the case, and

I am so grateful that I got the chance to survive something that could have ended up very differently. My daughter needs me, her mother, even on my worst days. Even when my OCD symptoms flare up. Even when I make parenting mistakes. Even when I dislike myself. Even when I am not sure whether I am providing her with the best care or making the best decisions for her. She needs me. Because I am her mom and she is my daughter and because I know she will always love me.

Two years later, I still fight for her, and when I'm feeling low, when the darkness momentarily creeps in and it feels hard to live for myself, I live for her. On days when I'm too tired or feel like giving up, I think back to my rock bottom, and it makes me want to keep rising. I fight harder on those days. And sometimes if I get exhausted and don't want to fight for myself, those are the times I fight for my daughter and my husband and all my loved ones. I have worked to accept and love myself and talk in a positive voice. And most important, I realize life would be much worse without me in it. I live my life most days through CBT and not by what thoughts and feelings are going through my head but what I can control and do that given day. This involves lots of bonding time with my daughter and fun activities that I plan for the two of us together. Some are for myself too—to get out of my own head—cycling, classes, yoga, meditation, therapy, playing tennis, socializing with adults, or starting my own business.

I share my story because I want to give anyone hope who may need it so desperately right now. Hope that things will improve. Hope that no matter how low you are feeling right now about yourself and your baby, those feelings will pass. That anxious thoughts and feelings about yourself or your baby don't make you a monster at all.

They. Are. Just. Thoughts.

It is not your fault, and you should not feel guilty. Above all, please don't feel bad or embarrassed to ask for help. Looking back at my situation, I'm so thankful I spoke up when I did and asked for help. It took some time and definitely lots of patience to begin healing. And even now I still need to hope and be patient that things will continue to improve. Surround yourself with a lot of supportive people who can continue to lift you up. Because let's be honest—being a parent is very hard work even without the burden of mental illness.

Today I feel so lucky. I am the stay-at-home mom I'd dreamed of being back when I was trying to get pregnant and then as my daughter was growing inside of me. I am her sole caretaker during the day, and my husband helps at night and on the weekends. As a toddler, my daughter is so sweet, smart, social, beautiful, and fun. And she has that extra silliness, like her mama. Most days you can find us dancing around the house and laughing uncontrollably. We have matching pajama nights and love to go out for adventures in the city, and my little girl has taught me what it is like to be completely selfless. When I look at her and she smiles and I see the twinkle in her eye, I know my journey was worth it. When she runs into my arms excitedly yelling, "Mommy, Mommy!" I know that this is who I was meant to be. At bedtime or when she gets up in the middle of the night or when she is sick, she only wants me, and she lays on me for hours, our two hearts beating as one. We have already made so many amazing memories together these past two years, and I just keep dreaming about the future together and what it will be like as we grow older together. We have so much fun together and as a family of three.

But then there is the looming question: Will we expand our family? It's asked by others, and it's my own internal question. My answer is that it is most important for my daughter to have a healthy mom. I do feel sad when I think that she may never have a sibling, but I am confident that she will understand when she is old enough. And if I do have another child, I will stay on medication throughout my pregnancy and beyond and do things completely differently this time around. I now know how important it is for both the mother and the baby to be healthy, and that means physical and mental health.

I will arm myself during pregnancy and have a plan for afterward.

But even with all of this knowledge, my husband and I have yet to make up our minds about whether to expand our family. I'm also open to other avenues to growing our family. We've thought about adoption and thought about surrogacy, and I'm grateful that these options exist for us to explore and plan to explore even further down the road. In my heart of hearts, I would love to have another child, but I'm just so nervous that my severe postpartum mental-health issues would flare up again.

I am being as honest as I can when I say that if that is the case, then I don't think it's worth it.

Not only do I have my daughter, but I already have a son. He just happens to be a canine beagle mix who is best friends with my daughter and with whom I am madly in love as well.

Because I do not know what our future holds, I've really made sure to take in all of my daughter's baby moments over the last couple of years: every milestone and memory has that much more weight, as I know that I may never be able to experience them again as a mom. And after all I've been through, it truly makes me appreciate every second of my time on earth with my daughter that much more. The silver lining to this battle I've fought is knowing I appreciate her and our time together that much more and am so grateful. I'm usually moving so quickly through life, but with her, I'm able to slow down and savor the moments.

I am beyond grateful for my little imperfect but yet oh-so-perfect family that I cherish with my entire heart. I am so grateful for my support system of unbelievable family members and friends who helped me to get here today. I am so thankful for my husband, for sticking by me, loving me, being my best friend, being a great father, and believing in me. My story is, and will always be, dedicated to my daughter. You will always be my source of light and hope. I love watching you grow and taking care of you, and you are my shining star. It brings me so much joy and a sense of accomplishment to see you so happy and thriving. The bond we have worked so hard to grow is truly unbreakable. We will always be best friends. This I am certain of. I love you lots, Charley Paige.

KENNY, THIRTY-SEVEN YEARS OLD

Living through a trauma is like becoming unstuck in time. A mere moment can seem endless, and months can pass by in the blink of an eye. Key events can be remembered in the sharpest of detail or, conversely, be a spot of utter blankness. Life occurs as if it is a warped record, causing the needle to bounce randomly from one track to another, never completing a song in its entirety.

When our second child, our son, Beau, was born, I became unstuck in time.

I can remember receiving the call that Becca, my beloved wife, was going to go into surgery and that I needed to drop everything and get to the hospital. This happened on a Thursday, while I was at work, and happened to be in the middle of an important meeting with a US senator. There was no time to change out of the navy blue suit I was wearing, so I laughed as I realized that I would be, unexpectedly, very well dressed when first meeting my new son.

I can remember greeting Becca at the hospital, just as she was to be rolled away for presurgery prep. We didn't have much time to talk, but in the few moments we did have, she asked me to wear her bright purple socks, for good luck, as they'd made her take them off before going into the OR. I then donned the surgery-room outfit—a white disposable jumpsuit; white, gauzy booties; a large, white hair cap; and a surgical mask—and waited until they brought me back to be with Becca while they prepared to open her up and retrieve our baby.

I can remember the mix of both drug-induced euphoria and intense fear in my Becca's eyes as I sat with her during the surgery. When our son, Alexander Beau (or "Beau," as we affectionately call him), was officially born at 4:11 P.M., we both laughed at the coincidence, as Becca's birthday is April 11. 4/11.

I can remember holding my son and bringing him close to my wife, who was still on the table as they worked to put everything back into place and sew her up. We softly sang a little family song to him and cried. He was perfect.

From that point on, my memories become much less clear and much more jagged.

There was a social worker who asked Becca some questions about how she was feeling, emotionally, and some questions were raised about potential postpartum depression. Despite any concerns, real or perceived, we—wife, baby, husband, disease—were sent home.

A week later, during the bris, an event that brings family and close friends together in celebration of the birth of a boy in the Jewish faith, Becca refused to leave our bedroom after the ceremony. Instead, she huddled under the covers, staying in bed all day with Beau, allowing only our postpartum doula, her sister, and her best friend in the room with her. The rest of our family and friends weren't able to grasp what was happening.

Then it got so much worse. Though this unstuck period is a blur, it's also more emotionally evocative than any other in my life. It is vague but intense, all at the same time, like the sound of that record playing, but so loudly that the speakers quake, obscuring the music, so that it's just noise. Loud, unsettling, uncomfortable noise.

I remember moments of extreme panic and fear.

Discovering Becca was intentionally hurting herself.

Having to forcibly open a bathroom door and restrain her from causing more harm to herself.

Moments when Becca would be in a near-comatose state, including at Thanksgiving, when she sat on a leather chair, head in hands, not taking a single bite of food, barely speaking to anyone. I sat beside her, balancing my own untouched plate of Thanksgiving fixings, while gently rocking the car seat that held our sleeping newborn, Beau.

There were psychiatric consultations, medicines prescribed, and then talks of a higher level of care at specialized facilities in other states.

There was the afternoon, after Becca and I had taken an exceedingly rare break from everything to see a movie, when we'd come home to discover that Beau felt like he was burning up. Off to the emergency room the three of us went, and while our son was being admitted for a bad case of RSV, Becca became faint and was also admitted to the ER for tests and observation. There they were, mother and son, in a makeshift emergency-room suite for two.

That's when our deafening record stopped playing abruptly, with just one, final, ear-piercing screech.

There is more—so much more—and I know this because I lived it, but trying to retell the story in full detail would be like trying to finish a complicated puzzle without the picture showing what the thousands of pieces are intended to create.

What I do know, with extreme, high-definition clarity, is that the experience of Becca's severe prenatal and postpartum depression and the collateral damage have forever changed us. As her primary caretaker, I know that, aside from Becca, this experience has impacted me the most. I do not say this selfishly; I say it honestly. It has been over five years since I became unstuck in time, and I am just now finding my own stability.

So, with all that being said, the idea of further expanding our family carries an immense amount of emotional baggage. And considerable fear.

It isn't fair. Not to my wife, not to my children, and neither even to me.

Our life, and the path we choose to take, should not be marred by events, terrible though they may be, that were not in our control or of our making. The decision to have another child should be made considering practical and emotional factors and not be ruled by fear.

It would be disingenuous to say that, for me, the fear is not the overwhelming factor at play when I try to reconcile my own feelings about expanding our family. Consider this: Following the birth of our son—which, on top of everything I have already mentioned, was compounded by a complicated surgery and concerns that, along with ominous mental-health factors, Becca might not be physically capable of safely carrying another child to term—this bitter brew of concerns compelled me to have a hasty vasectomy on a frigid, snowy morning in January 2014, just three months after Beau was born. In hindsight, it was a poorly thought-out, knee-jerk reaction.

These are the kinds of things that you do when you become unstuck in time.

Despite everything—the fear, the anxiety, the uncomfortable surgical procedure, the time spent out of the office, the therapy sessions, the hospitalizations, the anger, and the generally pervasive feeling of "This really sucks"—there was a period of time, specifically in 2017, during which I changed my mind. After years of saying "Absolutely not—there is no chance," I suddenly saw the scene that Becca had been seeing, on repeat, for years. A scene in which our family grew and joy grew along with it. I did not see it because she was pointing it out to me, but I saw it on my own.

Suddenly, and with steadfast conviction, I truly and desperately wanted to have another child. My proverbial switch flipped, and it flipped hard. This would be the B side of our record—which is, so often, the hidden gem.

I am not entirely sure where this came from, but I have my suspicions. Perhaps it was the fear of nearly losing Becca and then finally praising whatever higher power there might be that I did not. More likely, it was related to other outside stuff that was happening in our lives—namely, losing my father and being in the process of losing my mother within a year and a half. What I do know is that, like I said, it wasn't a decision based on the constant yearning Becca had expressed to me about having another child. I already knew her feelings, and until the switch suddenly flipped in me, I'd been immovable in my stance.

When I told Becca about my change of heart, she was, as I expected, elated. But as I kept reinforcing to her, this was not a decision I was making for her; it was a decision for myself. For us.

I can remember telling her, "Our children bring us so much joy. Adding to our family would only increase that joy!"

We had to consult fertility specialists, because, you know, the vasectomy. It was a whole ordeal. I was not easy or particularly supportive during the first round of IVF, when Becca was pumping herself with shots and hormones in preparation for an egg retrieval, and I was going to be sedated so they could surgically remove sperm from my body. To be perfectly honest, in retrospect, I was an awful partner. It was an incredibly emotionally charged situation, and I felt utterly overloaded. This presented itself as a hair-trigger temper as well as unfounded resentment toward Becca that I was in this situation. I had gotten the vasectomy, and I had changed my mind, and yet she was the one I blamed for everything. I was angry at the world for our misfortune (for Becca's mental-health issues and for making my mother sick and for the weather), and because she is the person closest to me, Becca bore the brunt of this anger. And yet she still continued to take the shots and endure daily visits to the doctor for blood tests and ultrasounds. She did this all alone. The fact that the results of the initial round of IVF yielded one viable fertilized egg didn't help.

Following that process, I went from complete and utter devotion to the idea of having another baby to something akin to "No fucking way!" You can imagine the devastation this caused Becca. All she had wanted was for me to be on the same page with her—that is to say, completely dedicated to and enthusiastic about expanding our family. There I was, one day, promising that I was "one million percent all in!" The next day I was one million percent all out. We were both ping-ponging, emotionally.

Again, like other major decisions made while unstuck in time, this one was not necessarily well thought out. Not by me, at least. I'm not proud of this time, but this time is a chapter in our story.

As the dust settled over the failure of the first round of IVF and I was able to take stock of how I truly felt, I was no longer unstuck in time but stranded on a rickety boat that was violently rocking in the middle of a sea between waves of "Yes, let's do this" and waves of "I'm running for the hills!"

At some point, the winds shifted the waves enough so that Becca was able to assist me in disembarking from my now-leaking boat and going for a second round of IVF. Unlike the first go-around, we approached the second attempt as a team united. We went to each other's appointments and listened carefully to the recommendations from the specialists. We followed all of the directions ("Take this medicine" and "Do not have any drinks"). Everyone—Becca, me, the team of doctors—all felt that we were in a good position for success.

We were not successful. Despite a successful sperm and egg retrieval, they were able to create zero viable embryos.

It was devastating. I cannot begin to imagine how Becca truly felt, but I know it would be putting it lightly to say that the blow to her was delivered with the power of a heavyweight-boxing champion. As for me, I was flung back onto the boat of indecision, which had now sprung multiple leaks and was being buffeted by massive rogue waves of "I'm running for the hills!"

As time passed and I managed to plug some of the holes in that boat, the seas calmed, and I was able to notice that there was a sun and that it was shining. Instead of constantly feeling I was in danger of drowning, I was able to dangle my feet in the water and feel things on my own terms.

What I felt was that things will happen to us in life that we do not choose and that sometimes those things will be terrible. I felt, and feel, like my family got a raw deal. I did not choose for Becca and me to suffer the traumas we each endured. I would not wish that breed of pain on anyone. I did not choose to have two unsuccessful rounds of IVF, despite Becca's abundant fertility and my own chosen infertility—by way of said snipping.

I did not choose to become unstuck in time.

What I've realized is that while I feel happy and content with our family and don't feel the need to expand it, I recognize that Becca does not, or cannot, feel the same way. I recognize that while it is possible to feel one way, it is also possible to feel, without a doubt, that if Becca says to me that she wants to continue trying through IVF or to pursue adoption or to look seriously into any other means of expanding our family, I will be all in at one million percent. It is something I can easily and willingly get behind but not something I will choose if it is my own decision.

In the meantime, I'm perfectly happy to keep dangling my feet in the now-calm waters as time passes in its relatively normal course.

I am no longer unstuck in time, nor am I stuck on one particular path. I am on this ride and will keep going with Becca and my kids by my side. Where will the boat float us if I decide to let it roll with the tide and not paddle in one direction or another? I'm not sure, but I know that, no matter what, I'm not going anywhere. I don't think I'll ever feel the need to have another baby like Becca does, but I will work toward finding peace for our family once more.

I will cherish the vibrant life—the fortified ship—the collection of vinyl—that we've built.

I will buy us a new record.

I will let us finish our song.

9

❖ ❖

Holding the Keys

As I write this, another page has just blown, noiselessly, off of the proverbial calendar of life; 2019 is now upon us. Gleaming, white snow coats the trees outside of my house in a layer that is simultaneously both thin and sturdy. This is how I feel often. I am thin and sturdy, and sometimes I can even glisten. This combination confuses people; I no longer fit neatly into a category, as I am not a "sufferer," nor am I "healed."

It is now one of the coldest days of the year. I am inside, by the fire, and although my body is warm, and although I am safe, the familiar feeling of discomfort that has burrowed deep within my chest is making me squirm in my seat. It feels like a weight and like a burning, and it sits right by my sternum, with tentacle-like arms that stretch down into my stomach and around my back, grabbing at me. This is anxiety and fear, and at the moment it is because I am thinking about the baby. Or, more accurately, the "maybe baby."

Earlier this winter Kenny and I had another office visit with our fertility specialist, Dr. G. Most patients, I have learned, have one consult with their doctor in order to make a plan and then proceed with said plan while having sporadic phone check-ins with the physician or physician's assistants. This was my fourth in-person consult, an illustration of the torment that has undulated within me.

After our first round of IVF, during which time we made the one healthy embryo, I had made an appointment to speak to the doctor in person. I needed guidance, reassurance, hope. I remember rushing to him after a routine eye examination, and, as I sat across from him, everything looked a bit hazy through my recently dilated eyes. It was the perfect metaphor for how I was able to view the world. Nothing was ever clear.

"You were dealt a lousy hand," he said, with great sympathy. "You made great eggs, and then you overstimulated. Ken's sperm just were not mature. You went through everything you went through with the postpartum, and now you're trying again, and it just isn't fair."

As usual, I vocalized my feelings of gratitude and how, in many ways, it felt unfair for me to accept his kind words, as any self-pity would be supremely selfish. Unlike many of his patients, I had been able to conceive, carry, birth, and love two children of my own.

Once again, I apologized for my feelings of sorrow, as if they were not valid.

He validated my feelings and reminded me of all that I had endured.

"You have nothing to be sorry about."

He then wrote out an extremely kind, generous plan for round two and slid the paper across his large, mahogany desk so that I could read his offer to me.

My eyes had still not adjusted, and I could not read a word that he had written, but I cried, with gratitude, nonetheless.

At our most recent meeting, I, once again, apologized for "being a bother," and Dr. G dismissed my apology with a hug.

Kenny and I sat, side by side, across from the man who in many ways felt like the maker of my destiny, and I asked him, for a final time, what we should do.

"I know we have options. But if we really want to grow our family with another pregnancy, I'm worried. We have this one embryo," I choked out through my tears. "If we try to use it and it doesn't work, then we have nothing. I'm getting older, and my kids are getting older, and the longer we wait, the harder it will be. Should we try again? What are we supposed to do?"

I spouted off my worries and questions breathlessly.

His reply was not what I had expected.

"Let me ask you a question," Dr. G began. "Let's say that when you were on your way in to meet me, today you ran into a woman outside of the hospital, carrying a newborn baby. If she were able to provide you with medical records and you knew it'd be safe but she told you that she could not keep her baby and asked you if you would take him from her, would you do it?"

"In a heartbeat," I replied, without a pause. "In many ways, that would be my dream!"

He continued: "Here is what I'm going to tell you. We could try another cycle with you, and I could adjust the medicine again and see if we could make more embryos. I don't think you guys are going to have a different result, though. You could reverse the vasectomy, but I don't think you want that, either. You could use a sperm donor and make a baby with your egg and donor sperm. You could use an egg donor and a sperm donor and have an embryo implanted into you so that you would both be on a level playing field, so to speak. You can adopt an embryo and have that transferred into you."

My head was swimming. This entire journey had been about finding ways in which we could try to expand our family, exploring these choices, and then narrowing them down so that we could decide what, if anything, would be best for us. There had been such a great sense of hope that had come with the idea that we could, perhaps, have another baby. After years of mourning, I had been given (what felt like) a new lease on life.

But with every answer, new questions were arising, each one feeling like a little weight added to my already-burdened shoulders. With every new option presented to me, new doors were opening. But instead of this affording me promise, it only caused more turmoil. It feels selfish and ungrateful to admit this, but this is my truth.

It was as if, for all this time, I had been staring into the night sky, hoping to find my answer, somewhere, written in the stars. With each step of my exploration, I was handed what I thought was a telescope, a powerful tool that would allow me to see everything so much more clearly. But when peering through the glass lens, I realized, over and over again, that these instruments were not telescopes, but rather kaleidoscopes. Instead of a clear view of my trail of stars, I saw a cubist prism of light, each facet distorting the picture behind it, leaving me more confused than ever before.

My attention snapped back to the room, where my doctor was still speaking.

"Listen," Dr. G said, gearing up for his big finish. I prayed that it contained some sort of clear, finite answer. "I see how much you're suffering. You're crippled by this. And I see your husband and how painful this is for him, because all he wants is for you to be happy."

Kenny nodded in appreciative agreement.

"I also know that you have this one embryo frozen here, and it is, biologically, the sibling of your two kids. I know you, and I don't think you're going to be walking away from this. So I say we leave it up to God."

Ordinarily, physicians (or at least the physicians that I've seen) do not bring up the notion of a higher power, let alone talk about God during consultations. In many cases, this is because doctors are scientists and scientists rely on data and numbers and the things that we can understand and study and see. In most cases, this is because outside of religiously affiliated hospitals and clinics, some might consider the mention of "God" inappropriate. But we had developed a rapport with Dr. G that transcended the traditional level of doctor-patient propriety. After all, most physicians do not say the words *I am going to get you pregnant*.

He presented us with the one plan that he thought was best for *us*. When we were ready, we would call his office, and they would begin to track my natural and regular cycle. He would put me on some medication, but only a minimal amount (as opposed to an oral-contraceptive pill that would chemically dictate my cycle). He would give me progesterone to help support my uterine lining, which had gotten "thick and pillowy" during each of my IVF cycles thus far, as he reminded us that my "body knows what to do in terms of carrying a pregnancy." During the time of my natural ovulation, he would do an embryo transfer on me, manually inserting our frozen embryo into my uterus, and we would see what happened. Because of the PGS, the chance that the pregnancy would take, with the embryo implanting, would be better than 50 percent (the actual number being significantly higher than that), but we all knew better than to rely on statistics.

"What is meant to be will be," Dr. G said, folding his hands in front of him, a sign of his conviction.

In that moment, my initial reaction was surprise. This was a doctor who could benefit greatly from having me try again, in some other way, to make and carry a baby. With another round or two of IVF, he would be making a lot more money, and his odds of achieving a successful pregnancy for me would go up exponentially. I was the patient that *should* get pregnant, and yet that's not what he suggested. He suggested what he believed was right.

Kenny, who had remained quiet during the appointment—and, in truth, during the weeks and months leading up to the appointment—spoke up with a level of assertive confidence that I had not heard from him surrounding the baby topic in a long time.

"I agree with you 100 percent," he told the doctor.

Surprised, I was, once more.

While this plan made me nervous in its tenuousness, their resolve was incredibly reassuring.

And more than anything, it was a plan.

As we start to settle into this new year, with 2019 undoubtedly poised to bring us new opportunities and challenges and perspectives, it is clear to me just how far I've come. It might not look like it from the outside, but I feel it, profoundly. You see, having another baby, by any means, would be taking a trip down a very new, potentially arduous path. I had been having enough trouble trying to decide whether to start the trek, but, what with all of the options and suboptions, I don't even know which direction to begin. I have my hiking boots on, but my hands are shaking too badly to be able to tie them. I hold a compass in my hands, but I am spinning around so quickly—so mercilessly—that it cannot orient itself; it provides me with no sense of direction. Each night, I look to the night sky to find the North Star and see nothing but opaque grayness. I realize, now, that I will not be able to count on another other person or object or plan to decide my fate; I will have to make this choice myself.

We so often talk about the things we carry. They are the things that we hold with us each day, present with every breath we take as we move through our lives. For me, the things I carry are colored (if not dominated) by that which I may never carry again.

The thing I carry is an emptiness.

Presumably, something being removed from one's shoulders (or plate or life or whatever metaphor you choose) should lighten the load. But for me, nothing about my yearning for another baby (and, as of this point, not having one) felt freeing. I did not feel liberated, nor did I feel lighter. I felt weighed down by something that has no tangible weight to it. I was encumbered by something that cannot be seen or heard or touched.

The thing I carried was the person I may never know.

And most troubling of all, the person who was controlling my life the most during these days was one who does not even exist.

This may seem hyperbolic or even wrong. Of course, in my daily life I am overwhelmed with love for my children, husband, family members, and friends. I am tasked with responsibilities to keep their schedules, tummies, and hearts full. But if I am speaking my most profound of truths, nearly everything and *everything* I do is, somehow, connected to this baby. Whether I will have a baby. If I should have a baby or if I should not have a baby. What this activity or this day or this life would look like with a baby in my arms. What would it be like to have another daughter? Another son? What would this person be named? Who would this person be?

Or what life would look like without one.

My mind returns to the image of the castle and the moat and the baby calling to me. I am standing there, stronger and more educated, but still on the other side.

The baby is still calling out to me, its voice as strong as ever. The baby looks different now; perhaps it is more realistic. It cries for me, and my heart aches, but when I look down at my waist, I see something. Something that was not there before.

It is not a big, pregnant belly; nor is it even a burgeoning bump. It is a tool belt. On it is a thick, braided piece of rope, expertly knotted. There is a life vest hanging from a metal clip. There is a mini tackle box filled with bait to throw far enough to distract the creatures that might bite and chomp and gnarl at me. There is a satchel filled with used-up needles and empty pill bottles and edge-worn pamphlets, and they remind me of just how far I've come.

My head snaps back up to attention.

"Please, Mommy! Please find me!" cries the baby.

"I'm still trying, Baby!" I scream across the water. "I see you! Mommy is trying to figure this out, Baby! I promise you, Mommy is trying!"

Mommy.

Baby.

It never stops breaking my heart.

And suddenly, all the world goes quiet.

In front of me, I can see the baby, far away, across the not-so-treacherous moat. The baby's face is red and soaked with hot tears. Its arms are reaching out toward me.

I step one foot closer to the baby, my right leg now in front of my left, but before I grab my rope to try to launch across the divide, I put all of my weight onto that foot and use it to propel me as I pivot my body. My left foot is now in front of me, and I'm facing all that was once at my back.

At the horizon line in the distance, I see the darkness of my past. I can make out the image of the black clouds and the cold rain and the giant pieces of hail falling from the sky.

I got through that. I survived.

In front of the darkness, I see a line of people. They are my doctors. My treatment team members. My friends. My tribe.

I see my parents.

They are standing there, staring at me, never breaking my gaze.

These people have my back.

And right in front of me, I see Kenny and Belle and Beau. Their arms are linked together, stronger than any man-made fortress or any stone castle. With his free arm, Kenny reaches out his hand. I stare at their faces, one by one.

Belle's heart-shaped face, and the glow that radiates from within her, makes my breath catch in my chest. Beau's blue eyes shine, and he smiles at me with such love, and my eyes well up with tears.

And then there is Kenny. My knight. He sees me there, standing at the edge of the precarious water below, weighed down by my cumbersome tool belt, and he does not flinch. He nods at me, still holding out his hand, just has he always has.

The world is quiet except for the pounding of my beating heart. I can hear it drumming loudly in my ears.

I know that behind me the baby is still there, crying, and begging for me to come to the rescue.

"I'm trying, Baby." I whisper once again, so softly that only I can hear.

Finally, I make a move.

This time it is not a pivot but a real step. I step forward, toward my family, and I take Kenny's hand and allow him to squeeze my own in his gentle but solid grasp.

Squeeze-squeeze-squeeze. He is saying, "I love you."

Squeeze-squeeze-squeeze-squeeze. "I love you, too."

The four of us are linked—impenetrable.

I nod, almost imperceptibly, and we all take a step forward, together, in perfect unison.

While the decision about another baby might ultimately be mine, it is one that we will make together. And no matter what I decide, we will tackle it all as a team. The team that we have worked so hard to build and to fortify.

I am still a tree. Some days I stand tall, boasting my vibrant leaves and lengthy branches. Some days I sway in the wind, in one direction and then another. Back and forth. Back and forth. Some days I feel so solid, silently counting the rings that have grown inside of me. Some days I feel so hollow.

But I am a tree, still standing, with roots deeper than I thought possible.

I do not know how many pieces of fruit my branches will grow, but I know that my fruit is more delicious and more sweet and more spectacular than I ever could have imagined.

I am a tree. I carry strength. I carry my family. I carry babies. I carry fruit.

Here I stand.

Here I grow.

Notes

CHAPTER 1

1. Centers for Disease Control and Prevention, "Prevalence of Self-Reported Postpartum Depressive Symptoms—17 States, 2004–2005," *Morbidity and Mortality Weekly Report* 57, no. 14, (2008): 361–66, https://www.cdc.gov/mmwr/preview/mmwrhtml/mm5714a1.htm; Katherine Stone, "How Many Women Get Postpartum Depression? The Statistics on PPD," *Postpartum Progress*, April 10, 2008, https://postpartumprogress.com/how-many-women-get-postpartum-depression-the-statistics-on-ppd.

2. Our current understanding of Zyprexa is that the dosage breastfeeding babies receive through their mothers is so low as to often be completely undetectable. See *MotherToBaby*, "Olanzapine (Zyprexa®)," August 1, 2018, https://mothertobaby.org/fact-sheets/olanzapine/.

3. Bret Weinstein, "Bret Weinstein," interview by Dax Shepard and Monica Padman, *Armchair Expert*, podcast audio, January 24, 2019, https://armchairexpertpod.com/pods/bret-weinstein.

4. My January 30, 2019, tweet to @DaxShepard, and his response, https://twitter.com/daxshepard/status/1090655901063598080; and here's my exchange that same day with @BretWeinstein, https://twitter.com/BretWeinstein/status/1090712650978254848.

CHAPTER 3

1. Rachel A. Becker, "How Did a Quail Chick Hatch from a Supermarket Egg?" *National Geographic*, March 16, 2016, https://www.nationalgeographic.com/people-and-culture/food/the-plate/2016/03/16/how-did-a-quail-chick-hatch-from-a-supermarket-egg/.

2. Division of Nutrition, Physical Activity, and Obesity, National Center for Chronic Disease Prevention and Health Promotion, "Body Mass Index (BMI)," Centers for Disease Control and Prevention, last reviewed May 15, 2015, https://www.cdc.gov/healthyweight/assessing/bmi/index.html.

3. US Food and Drug Administration, "Pregnancy and Lactation Labeling (Drugs) Final Rule," December 3, 2014, https://www.fda.gov/drugs/development approvalprocess/developmentresources/labeling/ucm093307.htm.

4. Emphasis mine. US Department of Health and Human Services, "FDA Pregnancy Categories," last updated May 29, 2019, https://chemm.nlm.nih.gov/pregnancycategories.htm.

5. "Klonopin: Dosage," *RxList*, last reviewed December 20, 2017, https://www.rxlist.com/klonopin-drug.htm#dosage.

6. Mayo Clinic Staff, "Antidepressants: Safe during Pregnancy?" Mayo Clinic (website), February 28, 2018, https://www.mayoclinic.org/healthy-lifestyle/preg nancy-week-by-week/in-depth/antidepressants/art-20046420.

7. Liz Tracy, "Why I Stayed on Antidepressants while Pregnant and Nursing," *The Atlantic*, May 22, 2017, https://www.theatlantic.com/health/archive/2017/05/deciding-to-stay-on-antidepressants-while-pregnant-and-nursing/527613/.

CHAPTER 4

1. See, for example, Illinois Department of Public Health, "Facts about Postpartum Depression," Women's Health, visited May 30, 2019, http://www.idph.state.il.us/about/womenshealth/factsheets/pdpress.htm.

2. Rebecca Fox Starr, *Beyond the Baby Blues: Anxiety and Depression During and After Pregnancy* (Lanham, MD: Rowman & Littlefield, 2018), 25.

3. Preeclampsia is a potentially fatal physical disorder occurring only during pregnancy and in the postpartum period, characterized by high blood pressure, among other symptoms. It affects at least 5–8 percent of all pregnancies. Learn more at the Preeclampsia Foundation, "About Preeclampsia," last updated January 3, 2019, https://www.preeclampsia.org/health-information/about-preeclampsia.

4. Karen R. Kleiman, *What Am I Thinking? Having a Baby after Postpartum Depression* (N.p.: Xlibris, 2005), 13.

5. American Psychological Association, "What Is Postpartum Depression & Anxiety?" visited May 30, 2019, https://www.apa.org/pi/women/resources/reports/postpartum-depression.aspx.

6. Fox Starr, *Beyond the Baby Blues*, 28.

7. Madeline R. Vann, "Will Postpartum Depression Return the Second Time Around?" *Everyday Health*, last updated June 7, 2011, https://www.every dayhealth.com/depression/will-postpartum-depression-return-the-second-time-around.aspx.

8. Ibid.

9. Fox Starr, *Beyond the Baby Blues*, 30–31, with internal quotations from Kimberly A. Yonkers et al., "The Management of Depression during Pregnancy: A Report from the American Psychiatric Association and the American College of Obstetricians and Gynecologists," *Obstetrics and Gynecology* 114, no. 3 (2009): 703–13, doi.org/10.1097/AOG.0b013e3181ba0632.

10. Christine Dunkel Schetter and Lynlee Tanner, "Anxiety, Depression and Stress in Pregnancy: Implications for Mothers, Children, Research, and Practice," *Current Opinion in Psychiatry* 25, no. 2 (2012): 141–48, doi:10.1097/YCO.0b013e3283503680.

11. Fox Starr, *Beyond the Baby Blues*.

CHAPTER 5

1. Cheryl Wetzstein, "Study: Families Trending toward Open Adoptions," *Washington Times*, March 21, 2012, https://www.washingtontimes.com/news/2012/mar/21/study-families-trending-toward-open-adoptions/.

2. Ibid.

3. Amy's is one of several stories shared in Katherine Stone, "7 Postpartum Depression Survivors Share Their Stories of Having More Children," *Postpartum Progress*, February 12, 2012, https://postpartumprogress.com/7-postpartum -depression-survivors-share-their-stories-of-having-more-children.

4. From the title banner of Amy Brannan's blog, *Living Life Joyously*, found at https://livinglifejoyously.blogspot.com/.

5. Amy Brannan, "A First for Me Today," *Living Life Joyously*, June 10, 2010, https://livinglifejoyously.blogspot.com/2010/06/first-for-me-today.html.

6. Amy Brannan, "Profile Online Now," *Living Life Joyously*, January 3, 2011, https://livinglifejoyously.blogspot.com/2011/01/profile-online-now.html.

7. Amy Brannan, "Loss and Fear," *Living Life Joyously*, January 25, 2011, https://livinglifejoyously.blogspot.com/2011/01/loss-and-fear.html.

8. Amy Brannan, "The Raw Truth That I Deal with Daily," *Living Life Joyously*, January 4, 2011, https://livinglifejoyously.blogspot.com/2011/01/raw-truth -that-i-deal-with-daily.html.

9. Amy Brannan, "More Babies," *Living Life Joyously*, May 6, 2011, https://livinglifejoyously.blogspot.com/2011/05/more-babies.html.

10. As quoted in Stone, "7 Postpartum Depression Survivors Share Their Stories."

11. Amy Brannan, "It's Been a Long Time—So Much Has Happened," *Living Life Joyously*, August 4, 2013, https://livinglifejoyously.blogspot.com/2013/08/its-been-long-time-so-much-has-happened.html.

12. Amy Brannan, "Almost 1 Year," *Living Life Joyously*, August 20, 2013, https://livinglifejoyously.blogspot.com/2013/08/one-year-old.html.

13. Amy Brannan, "A Year Ago Today, Our World Turned Upside Down," *Living Life Joyously*, February 9, 2018, https://livinglifejoyously.blogspot.com/2018/02/a-year-ago-today-our-world-turned.html.

14. Karen J. Foli, "Depression in Adoptive Parents: A Model of Understanding through Grounded Theory," *Western Journal of Nursing Research* 32, no. 3 (2009): 379–400, doi:10.1177/0193945909351299.

15. Ibid.

16. Foli's researched described in Amanda MacMillan, "Post-adoption Depression: How to Manage This Difficult Side Effect of a Happy Event," Seleni Institute, March 16, 2018, https://www.seleni.org/advice-support/2018/3/16/post-adoption-depression. See also Amy Patterson Neubert, "Expectations, Exhaustion Can Lead Mothers to Post-adoption Stress," Purdue University, University News Service, March 22, 2012, https://www.purdue.edu/newsroom/research/2012/1203 22FoliResearch.html.

17. Sarah L. Mott et al., "Depression and Anxiety among Postpartum and Adoptive Mothers," *Archives of Women's Mental Health* 14, no. 4 (August 2011): 335, doi:10.1007/s00737-011-0227-1, https://www.ncbi.nlm.nih.gov/pmc/articles/PMC3433270/.

CHAPTER 6

1. Fox Starr, *Beyond the Baby Blues*, 77–78.

2. Alexandria Campbell, "15 Reasons to Opt for a Surrogate," *Babygaga*, February 7, 2017, https://www.babygaga.com/15-reasons-to-opt-for-a-surrogate/.

3. Natalia Lusinski, "6 Medical Reasons to Use a Surrogate," *Bustle*, June 21, 2017, https://www.bustle.com/p/6-medical-reasons-to-use-a-surrogate-65848.

4. WebMD, "Using a Surrogate Mother: What You Need to Know," reviewed September 7, 2017, https://www.webmd.com/infertility-and-reproduction/guide/using-surrogate-mother#1.

5. Susan Imrie and Vasanti Jadva, "The Long-Term Experiences of Surrogates: Relationships and Contact with Surrogacy Families in Genetic and Gestational Surrogacy Arrangements," *Reproductive BioMedicine Online* 29, no. 4 (2014): 424–35, doi:10.1016/j.rbmo.2014.06.004.

6. Mark P. Trolice, "Surrogacy in the USA—Is It Legal in All 50 States? History," *Babygest*, January 25, 2019, https://wearesurrogacy.com/united-states/#history.

7. WebMD, "Using a Surrogate Mother."

8. Council for Responsible Genetics, "About CRG," visited June 2, 2019, http://www.councilforresponsiblegenetics.org/Help/About.aspx; and Magdalina Gugucheva, *Surrogacy in America* (Cambridge, MA: Council for Responsible Genetics, 2010), http://www.councilforresponsiblegenetics.org/pageDocuments/KAEVEJ0A1M.pdf.

9. For more information on US law concerning surrogacy agreements, by state, visit *ARTparenting*, https://www.artparenting.com/surrogacy-agreements .html.

10. Lisa Marie Vari, "Gestational Surrogate Requirements in Pennsylvania," Lisa Marie Vari & Associates, P.C. (website), May 11, 2018, https://www.pafamily lawyers.com/gestational-surrogate-requirements-in-pennsylvania/.

11. MrsBraun, "Postpartum Depression Leads to Finding a Surrogate—Here's My Story," Adoption, *The Bump*, August 2012, https://forums.thebump.com/dis cussion/8435746/postpartum-depression-leads-to-finding-a-surrogate-heres-my -story.

12. Ibid.

13. Ibid.

14. Ibid.

15. MrsBraun, "Crazy Question—Anyone Here Use a Surrogate??" Babies on the Brain, *The Bump*, August 2012, https://forums.thebump.com/discussion/ 8435808/crazy-question-anyone-here-use-a-surrogate.

16. Ibid.

17. MrsBraun, "Random—Would You Name Your Child After Your Surro-gate??" Parenting, *The Bump*, August 2012, https://forums.thebump.com/discus sion/8441208/random-would-you-name-your-child-after-your-surrogate.

18. Ibid.

19. Ibid.

20. Ibid.

21. Christine uses the handle @storkstories.

22. Michelle uses the handle @michellegriffindoula.

Bibliography

American Psychological Association. "What Is Postpartum Depression & Anxiety?" Visited May 30, 2019. https://www.apa.org/pi/women/resources/reports/postpartum-depression.aspx.

Becker, Rachel A. "How Did a Quail Chick Hatch from a Supermarket Egg?" *National Geographic*. March 16, 2016. https://www.nationalgeographic.com/people-and-culture/food/the-plate/2016/03/16/how-did-a-quail-chick-hatch-from-a-supermarket-egg/.

Brannan, Amy. "Almost 1 Year." *Living Life Joyously*. August 20, 2013. https://livinglifejoyously.blogspot.com/2013/08/one-year-old.html.

———. "A First for Me Today." *Living Life Joyously*. June 10, 2010. https://livinglifejoyously.blogspot.com/2010/06/first-for-me-today.html.

———. "It's Been a Long Time—So Much Has Happened." *Living Life Joyously*. August 4, 2013. https://livinglifejoyously.blogspot.com/2013/08/its-been-long-time-so-much-has-happened.html.

———. "Loss and Fear." *Living Life Joyously*. January 25, 2011. https://livinglifejoyously.blogspot.com/2011/.

———. "More Babies." *Living Life Joyously*. May 6, 2011. https://livinglifejoyously.blogspot.com/2011/05/more-babies.html.

———. "Profile Online Now." *Living Life Joyously*. January 3, 2011. https://livinglifejoyously.blogspot.com/2011/01/profile-online-now.html.

———. "The Raw Truth That I Deal with Daily." *Living Life Joyously*. January 4, 2011. https://livinglifejoyously.blogspot.com/2011/01/raw-truth-that-i-deal-with-daily.html.

———. "A Year Ago Today, Our World Turned Upside Down." *Living Life Joyously*. February 9, 2018. https://livinglifejoyously.blogspot.com/2018/02/a-year-ago-today-our-world-turned.html.

Campbell, Alexandria. "15 Reasons to Opt for a Surrogate." *Babygaga*. February 7, 2017. https://www.babygaga.com/15-reasons-to-opt-for-a-surrogate/.

Centers for Disease Control and Prevention. "Prevalence of Self-Reported Postpartum Depressive Symptoms—17 States, 2004–2005." *Morbidity and Mortality Weekly Report* 57, no. 14 (2008): 361–66, https://www.cdc.gov/mmwr/preview/mmwrhtml/mm5714a1.htm.

Council for Responsible Genetics. "About CRG." Visited June 2, 2019. http://www.councilforresponsiblegenetics.org/Help/About.aspx.

Division of Nutrition, Physical Activity, and Obesity, National Center for Chronic Disease Prevention and Health Promotion. "Body Mass Index (BMI)." Centers for Disease Control and Prevention. Last reviewed May 15, 2015. https://www.cdc.gov/healthyweight/assessing/bmi/index.html.

Dunkel Schetter, Christine, and Lynlee Tanner. "Anxiety, Depression and Stress in Pregnancy: Implications for Mothers, Children, Research, and Practice." *Current Opinion in Psychiatry* 25, no. 2 (2012): 141–48. doi: 10.1097/YCO.0b013e3283503680.

Foli, Karen J. "Depression in Adoptive Parents: A Model of Understanding through Grounded Theory." *Western Journal of Nursing Research* 32, no. 3 (2009): 379–400. doi:10.1177/0193945909351299.

Fox Starr, Rebecca. *Beyond the Baby Blues: Anxiety and Depression During and After Pregnancy*. Lanham, MD: Rowman & Littlefield, 2018.

Gugucheva, Magdalina. *Surrogacy in America*. Cambridge, MA: Council for Responsible Genetics, 2010. http://www.councilforresponsiblegenetics.org/pageDocuments/KAEVEJ0A1M.pdf.

Illinois Department of Public Health. "Facts about Postpartum Depression." Women's Health. Visited May 30, 2019. http://www.idph.state.il.us/about/womenshealth/factsheets/pdpress.htm.

Imrie, Susan, and Vasanti Jadva. "The Long-Term Experiences of Surrogates: Relationships and Contact with Surrogacy Families in Genetic and Gestational Surrogacy Arrangements." *Reproductive BioMedicine Online* 29, no. 4 (2014): 424–35. doi:10.1016/j.rbmo.2014.06.004.

Kleiman, Karen R. *What Am I Thinking? Having a Baby after Postpartum Depression*. N.p.: Xlibris, 2005.

Lusinski, Natalia. "6 Medical Reasons to Use a Surrogate." *Bustle*. June 21, 2017. https://www.bustle.com/p/6-medical-reasons-to-use-a-surrogate-65848.

MacMillan, Amanda. "Post-adoption Depression: How to Manage This Difficult Side Effect of a Happy Event." Seleni Institute. March 16, 2018. https://www.seleni.org/advice-support/2018/3/16/post-adoption-depression.

Mayo Clinic Staff. "Antidepressants: Safe during Pregnancy?" Mayo Clinic (website). February 28, 2018. https://www.mayoclinic.org/healthy-lifestyle/pregnancy-week-by-week/in-depth/antidepressants/art-20046420.

MotherToBaby. "Olanzapine (Zyprexa®)." August 1, 2018. https://mothertobaby .org/fact-sheets/olanzapine/.

Mott, Sarah L., Crystal Edler Schiller, Jenny Gringer Richards, Michael W. O'Hara, and Scott Stuart. "Depression and Anxiety among Postpartum and Adoptive Mothers." *Archives of Women's Mental Health* 14, no. 4 (August 2011): 335–43. doi:10.1007/s00737-011-0227-1. https://www.ncbi.nlm.nih .gov/pmc/articles/PMC3433270/.

MrsBraun. "Crazy Question—Anyone Here Use a Surrogate??" Babies on the Brain. *The Bump*. August 2012. https://forums.thebump.com/discussion/8435808 /crazy-question-anyone-here-use-a-surrogate.

———. "Postpartum Depression Leads to Finding a Surrogate—Here's My Story." Adoption. *The Bump*. August 2012. https://forums.thebump.com/ discussion/8435746/postpartum-depression-leads-to-finding-a-surrogate-heres -my-story.

———. "Random—Would You Name Your Child After Your Surrogate??" Parenting. *The Bump*. August 2012. https://forums.thebump.com/discussion/ 8441208/random-would-you-name-your-child-after-your-surrogate.

Oliver, Mary. "Heavy." In *Thirst: Poems*, 53–54. Boston: Beacon Press, 2006.

Patterson Neubert, Amy. "Expectations, Exhaustion Can Lead Mothers to Post-adoption Stress." Purdue University, University News Service. March 22, 2012. https://www.purdue.edu/newsroom/research/2012/120322FoliResearch.html.

Preeclampsia Foundation. "About Preeclampsia." Last updated January 3, 2019. https://www.preeclampsia.org/health-information/about-preeclampsia.

RxList. "Klonopin: Dosage." Last reviewed December 20, 2017. https://www .rxlist.com/klonopin-drug.htm#dosage.

Stone, Katherine. "How Many Women Get Postpartum Depression? The Statistics on PPD." *Postpartum Progress*. April 10, 2008. https://postpartumprogress .com/how-many-women-get-postpartum-depression-the-statistics-on-ppd.

———. "7 Postpartum Depression Survivors Share Their Stories of Having More Children." *Postpartum Progress*. February 12, 2012. https://postpartum progress.com/7-postpartum-depression-survivors-share-their-stories-of-having -more-children.

Tracy, Liz. "Why I Stayed on Antidepressants while Pregnant and Nursing." *The Atlantic*. May 22, 2017. https://www.theatlantic.com/health/archive/2017/05/ deciding-to-stay-on-antidepressants-while-pregnant-and-nursing/527613/.

Trolice, Mark P. "Surrogacy in the USA—Is It Legal in All 50 States? History." *Babygest*. January 25, 2019. https://wearesurrogacy.com/united-states/#history.

US Department of Health and Human Services. "FDA Pregnancy Categories." Last updated May 29, 2019. https://chemm.nlm.nih.gov/pregnancycategories.htm.

US Food and Drug Administration. "Pregnancy and Lactation Labeling (Drugs) Final Rule." December 3, 2014. https://www.fda.gov/drugs/developmentap provalprocess/developmentresources/labeling/ucm093307.htm.

Vann, Madeline R. "Will Postpartum Depression Return the Second Time Around?" *Everyday Health*. Last updated June 7, 2011. https://www.every dayhealth.com/depression/will-postpartum-depression-return-the-second-time -around.aspx.

Vari, Lisa Marie. "Gestational Surrogate Requirements in Pennsylvania." Lisa Marie Vari & Associates, P.C. (website). May 11, 2018. https://www.pafamily lawyers.com/gestational-surrogate-requirements-in-pennsylvania/.

WebMD. "Using a Surrogate Mother: What You Need to Know." Reviewed September 7, 2017. https://www.webmd.com/infertility-and-reproduction/guide/ using-surrogate-mother#1.

Weinstein, Bret. "Bret Weinstein." Interview of Bret Weinstein with Dax Shepard and Monica Padman. *Armchair Expert*. Podcast audio. January 24, 2019. https:// armchairexpertpod.com/pods/bret-weinstein.

Wetzstein, Cheryl. "Study: Families Trending toward Open Adoptions." *Washington Times*. March 21, 2012. https://www.washingtontimes.com/news/2012/ mar/21/study-families-trending-toward-open-adoptions/.

Yonkers, Kimberly A., Katherine L. Wisner, Donna E. Stewart, Tim F. Oberlander, Diana L. Dell, Nada Stotland, Susan Ramin, Linda Chaudron, and Charles Lockwood. "The Management of Depression during Pregnancy: A Report from the American Psychiatric Association and the American College of Obstetricians and Gynecologists." *Obstetrics and Gynecology* 114, no. 3 (2009): 703–13. doi.org/10.1097/AOG.0b013e3181ba0632.

Index

About the Author

Rebecca Fox Starr is author, writer, blogger, mom, wife, and mental-health advocate. She created her internationally read blog, *Mommy, Ever After*, in 2010, and her first book, *Beyond the Baby Blues: Anxiety and Depression During and After Pregnancy*, was released in late 2017. Rebecca writes candidly about her life as mother, survivor, advocate, singer-songwriter, dance partier, and studded-shoe collector. Her story has been featured in the *New York Times* and *HuffPost*, on ABC News, and in all forms of media across the world. Rebecca writes and lives with her husband, daughter, son, and two dogs in the suburbs of Philadelphia. More about Rebecca can be found on her blog at http://mommyeverafter.com and on social media outlets @rebeccafoxstarr.